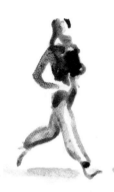

The Sensual Body

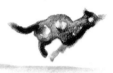

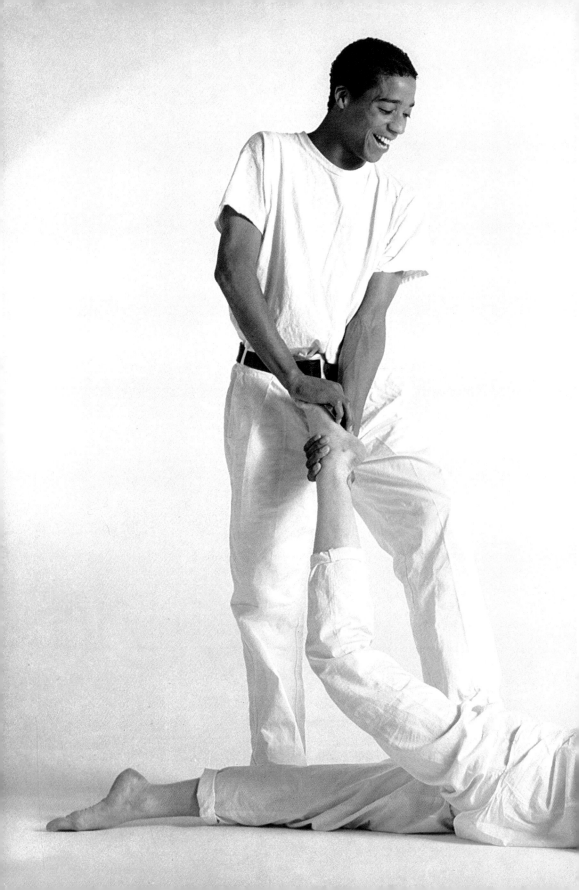

THE
SENSUAL
BODY

The Ultimate Guide to Body Awareness
and Self-fulfilment

by Lucy Lidell
and Sara Thomas

with Frankie Armstrong, Thérèse Van Cauwenberghe,
Peggy Harper, Denise Holmes, Barbara Karban, Denis Postle,
Franklin Sills, and Janaki Vincent

Photography by Fausto Dorelli

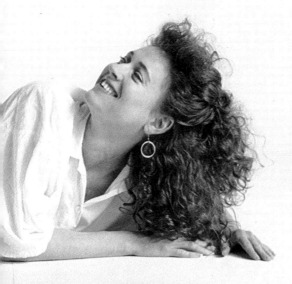

GUILD PUBLISHING LONDON

A GAIA ORIGINAL

Written by Lucy Lidell
and Sara Thomas (Massage)

with Frankie Armstrong, Darien Pritchard (Voicework)
Thérèse Van Cauwenberghe (Eutony)
Peggy Harper (African dance)
Denise Holmes (Aikido)
Barbara Karban (T'ai chi)
Denis Postle (Sensing, Relating)
Franklin Sills (Kum Nye)
Janaki Vincent (Running)

Photography by Fausto Dorelli
Assisted by Peter Warren

Editorial	Susan McKeever
Appendix	Barbara Kiser
Design	Margaret Sadler
Illustration	Pauline Hazelwood
Paintings	Barbara Karban
Direction	Joss Pearson
	Patrick Nugent
Production	Susan Walby

This edition published 1987 by Guild Publishing
by arrangement with Gaia Books Ltd and Unwin Hyman.

© 1987 Gaia Books Ltd., London

Printed in Spain by Artes Graficas Toledo S.A.
D.L. TO: 1967–1987

About this book

The Sensual Body is divided into three parts –
Prelude, Solowork, and *Partnerwork. Prelude* leads
you into the practical sections of the book: *Solowork*
which contains exercises and techniques for you to do
alone, and *Partnerwork,* which consists of exercises
for two people to do together. Whichever technique
you choose to learn, it's a good idea to begin by
reading the Introduction and *Prelude,* where the
theme of body awareness is introduced and where
practical advice is given relevant to all the techniques.

The Contributors

Sara Thomas has worked with holistic massage as
both teacher and practitioner for 10 years, and has
wide experience in other body and mind therapies.
Frankie Armstrong has been a folk singer since 1957,
and runs vocal workshops for both singers and
non-singers. She was assisted in her contribution by
Darien Pritchard. Thérèse Van Cauwenberghe
trained for 4 years with Gerda Alexander at the
Eutony School in Copenhagen. She has since taught
Eutony for 9 years in Brussels and London. *Peggy
Harper* is an African dance specialist who spent years
researching the subject at universities in Nigeria,
Ghana, and Sierra Leone. She has worked as a
choreographer in Nigeria, and was director of the
National Dance Company in Zimbabwe. *Denise
Holmes* has been teaching and training in Aikido for
4 years at the London Aikido Club. *Barbara Karban*
has been teaching T'ai chi for the past 9 years, and
also adds a special touch to the book with her
beautiful watercolours. *Denis Postle* is a
psychotherapist, counsellor, and writer of science
fiction. He has made many documentaries for
television on science and psychology-related themes.
Franklin Sills started studying Buddhist and Taoist
practices in 1973. He now teaches both Kum Nye and
Chi Kung in London and Devon. *Janaki Vincent,*
once a jazz dancer, is now a specialist counsellor in
Holistic Health and Psychic Massage.

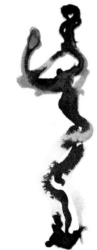

Note: *If you have any injuries
or chronic health problems,
consult your doctor before
attempting any of the
exercises, and observe the
cautions given in the book.*

To know who one is, an individual must
be aware of what he feels.

Alexander Lowen

Man has no body distinct from his soul.

William Blake

If you're an alive body, no-one can tell
you how to experience the world. And
no-one can tell you what truth is,
because you experience it for yourself.
The body does not lie.

Stanley Keleman

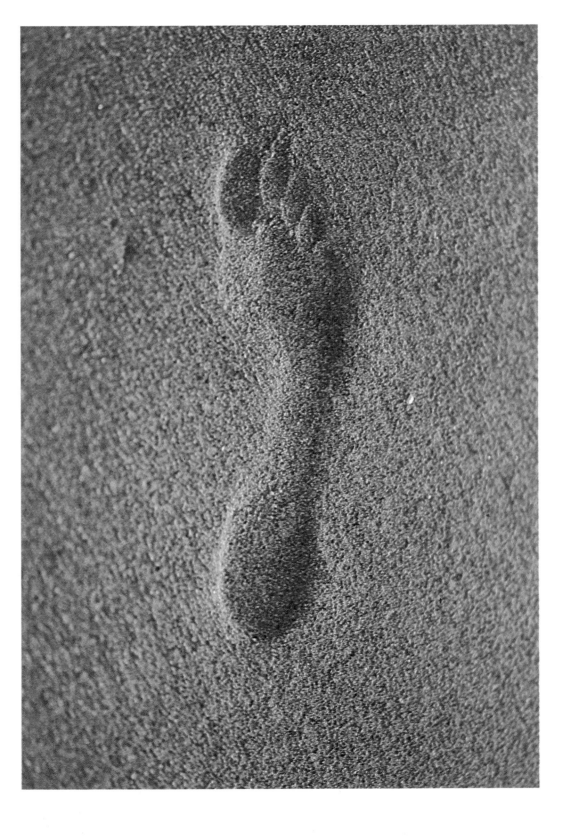

Contents

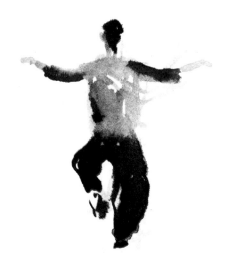

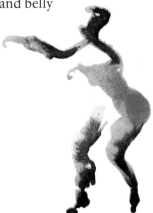

Introduction

All of us have known times when we felt totally at home in our bodies – vibrant, alive, assured, in touch with ourselves and aware of our sensual contact with the world around us. But for most these times are all too brief – enjoyed while on holiday, perhaps, only to fade soon after.

So what is body awareness and how can we retain the sense of aliveness and fulfilment it brings? Being aware of your body means having your attention fully in your body, living through your body, so that mind and body are united. Much of the time in adult life, our energy is predominantly in our heads, and we exist out of contact with parts of our bodies.

When you are fully aware of your body, you exist as one being, rejoicing in a feeling of harmony and integration. Your movements are free, spontaneous, co-ordinated and, like a small child or an animal, your perception is keen, your body charged with feeling. You possess an inner confidence, a sense of vitality, and a responsiveness to the world around you that are the essence of true sensuality.

When I first heard about body awareness, about the concept of "inhabiting" your body, I found the whole idea ridiculous. But then gradually, through doing yoga and, later, eutony, and through learning therapeutic massage, I began to understand what was meant. I started to realize when I was living too much in my head and to experience how very different I felt when I could sense my whole body. Giving people massage, I would be struck by the difference in energy, tone, and colour I could observe in different parts of their bodies. Slowly I began to see that the parts of which the person was aware were warmer and more alive, while those parts from which he or she was cut off felt, by contrast, cooler, sadder, and more toneless.

Contacting your body

Naturally, we all have some degree of body awareness, but few of us are fully aware of ourselves, and few make use of our full capacity for feeling.

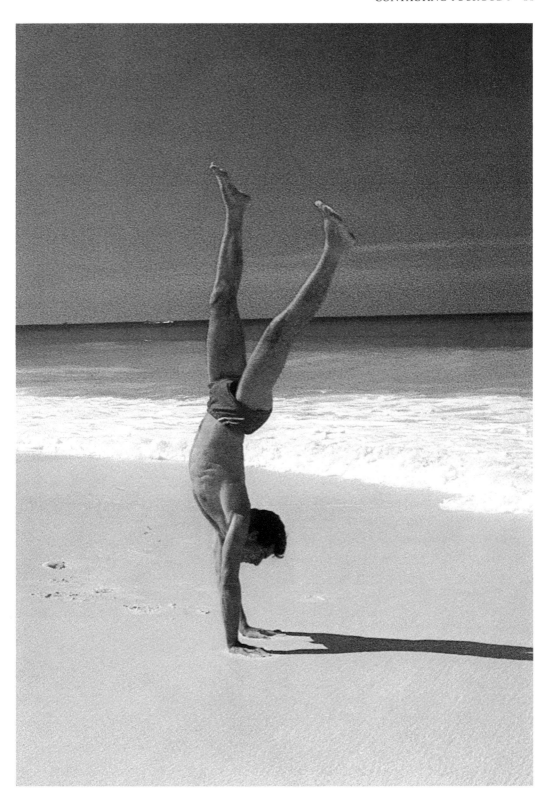

Most of us have an incomplete sense of our bodies – we may be strongly aware of our upper bodies, perhaps, but lack feeling in our legs and feet, or we may sense more in the right side of the body, say, than in the left.

One of the biggest obstacles in the way of understanding body awareness is that most of us don't realize how "dead" parts of our bodies are. We are used to the stiffness and tension we carry around and to relating to ourselves from the perspective of how we look rather than how we feel.

Trying this simple exercise will show you how your body feels at present. Sitting where you are or lying on the floor, close your eyes and feel your body touching the chair or the floor. Notice which parts of your body move as you breathe. Now allow your attention to wander slowly through your entire body from the inside. How much of yourself can you contact in this way? Are there parts that you can feel quite clearly and precisely and others that feel dull or blank? Do some parts feel lighter or larger or warmer than others? Can you feel the base of your spine...the back of your head...your toes? Is there a difference between your left and right sides? Are you aware of any areas of tension or sensations of heat or cold, tingling, pleasure or discomfort?

You may be surprised by what you find from this experiment. Many people discover that parts of the body feel blank or cut off. Others find that instead of really feeling a part of the body they tend to visualize it, using their inner eyes to travel around a picture of their bodies. Try the experiment again from time to time as you work through the book and see if anything changes.

Why is body awareness important?

Becoming more aware of your body quietens your mind and reawakens your senses. As you learn to stand and move in a more grounded way, with a strong sense of centre, your self-assurance grows. You cannot easily be thrown off balance or

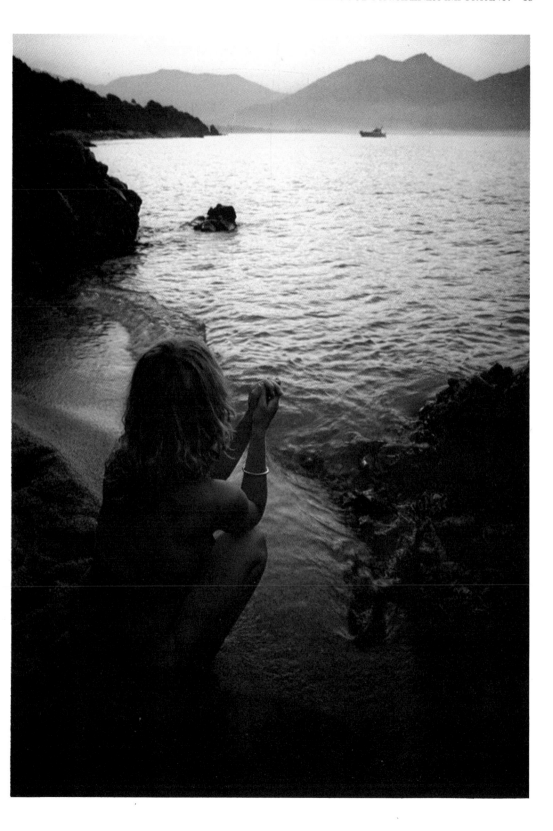

disoriented. With your mind and body acting as equal partners, you experience a new sense of wholeness. You feel more positive and alive, for your energy flows freely through your body.

The more you are in touch with your body, the more you know who you are and what you feel – for your sense of self is intimately linked with your awareness of your body.

Through regaining contact with your own centre and through learning not to withhold your feelings, you can relate more openly and honestly with your partner and friends. You may not always choose to express your feelings – but once you are aware of what you feel, as well as what you think, at least you can have the choice of deciding when it is appropriate to share how you feel.

"The feeling of identity stems from a feeling of contact with the body. To know who one is, an individual must be aware of what he feels. He should know the expression on his face, how he holds himself, and the way he moves. Without this awareness of bodily feeling and attitude, a person becomes split into a disembodied spirit and a disenchanted body."
Alexander Lowen

Body awareness and health

The body is intelligent – if we can only learn to understand its language, we can use what it tells us to stay relaxed and in tune with ourselves. For many of us it is only when we are in pain, when illness or injury affect a part of the body, that we are forced to pay attention, to reconnect with that aspect of ourselves that until now has been beyond our awareness.

Lack of contact with our bodies and feelings lies behind many illnesses. If we are not in harmony with ourselves, if we are deaf to the messages our body transmits, we run the risk of allowing the stress in our lives to develop past a level we can tolerate. Illness is often the only way we have of forcing ourselves to rest or slow down. Equally, if we endlessly suppress emotions such as anger or grief – or are unaware of even having them – the stress this causes will eventually affect us at a physical level, manifesting in all kinds of illnesses, both major and minor.

With greater awareness of your body, you can learn to take more responsibility for your own well-being. You can begin to listen when your body speaks, to open up a dialogue and heed its warnings,

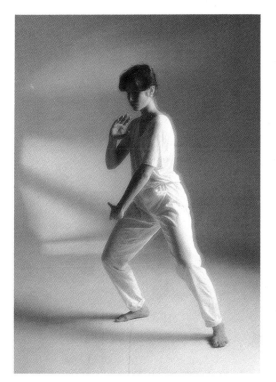

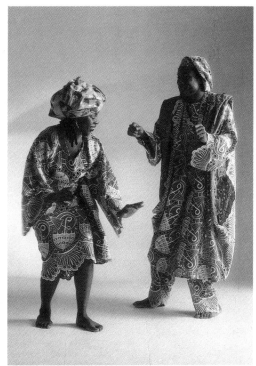

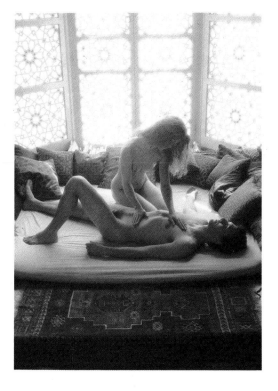

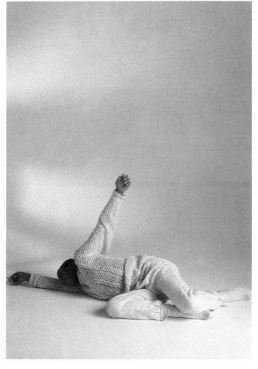

honour its needs. In time, you can come to know
what types of food really suit you, for example, which
kinds of people, or what causes you stress.

Ways to increase body awareness

Never before has there been so much interest in health
and fitness – in stress management, exercise, nutrition
and so on. But many types of exercise do little to
enhance body awareness – some may even serve to
widen the rift between body and mind. In any
competitive sport that focuses on winning, for instance,
there is an element of tension, diminishing its value as a
way of freeing the body. And in types of exercise done
to look good more than to feel good, the feeling life of
the body is largely ignored.

The disciplines introduced in this book have been
chosen specifically for their value in allowing you to
sense your body. Unlike most other physical
disciplines, they involve and integrate mind, body, and
spirit. Practised regularly, each can help you to make a
deeper contact with yourself, to dissolve stress and
tension and enhance your capacity for feeling. If you
find any of them particularly enjoyable, you can take
them further by going to classes. The disciplines chosen
represent a personal selection, however. They are by no
means the only ways to enhance body awareness –
others are described in the Appendix. And many
popular sports can serve to put you more in touch with
the body, once you understand the principles of body
awareness.

No-one can "give" you body awareness. The process
of reconnecting with your feelings and allowing
yourself to be more sensitive is one that each of us must
ultimately do for ourselves at our own pace, and in our
own time. But by experiencing how different life feels
when you get back in touch with the parts of yourself
that have lain dormant, you can gradually work
toward enjoying this feeling of vibrancy and sense of
unity more of the time, extending what you have
learned into your everyday life.

PRELUDE

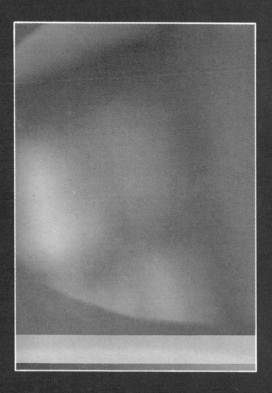

The deserted temple

If you travel outside Europe or the United States – in parts of South America, for instance, or in rural India or Africa – you cannot help being struck by the difference in the way people stand, move, and communicate with one another. Whilst in our more affluent urban cultures few people seem really at ease in their bodies, few display grace or fluidity in their movements, there, the majority move freely, confidently, rhythmically, at home in their bodies and aware of their personal space. When they speak, they talk with their whole beings, and at all ages people seem to retain a more solid sense of their bodies and their connection with the earth. The comparative awkwardness and stiffness of us Westerners is largely acquired, however, not innate. For most of us there was a time when we, too, lived and breathed and moved more naturally, more spontaneously, in tune with our feelings and with ourselves.

As small children, our bodies are our homes. From the moment we get up to the time we fall into bed, we are fully engrossed in our experience of life, excitedly exploring our capacities for balance, strength, and agility. We live in our senses, taking in and responding to the people and things we come across in our environment with directness and immediacy. When we are hurt, we cry with our whole bodies, when amused or excited, every muscle is involved. Our feelings are intense and wholehearted,

and once expressed, over and soon forgotten. We live in our own rhythm, our energy as yet unbounded by tension, our sensitivity undimmed.

As we grow up, however, much of this directness of perception may be lost and the feeling of comfort in our bodies superseded. Instead of unselfconsciously enjoying a sense of belonging inside our own skins, many of us start to become alienated from our physical selves. As we begin to compare ourselves with others, we may start to distance ourselves from our bodies, to feel awkward or uneasy about the way we look, to criticize our sizes or shapes. The body that was once for us a temple, a sanctuary of safety and joy, is gradually deserted as more and more we learn to live in our heads, to develop an inner hollowness. Though from the outside we may appear to be fine, inside the gap is widening between how we act and how we really feel. Slowly the body that once felt like home may begin to tense and stiffen. While as children we breathed freely and moved with natural grace and co-ordination, now our movements may be mechanical, may lack rhythm and harmony.

This chapter explores the reasons why you may vacate your natural home and lose awareness of your body so that you can better understand your own individual history and see what you can do to redeem the sense of wholeness and unity you once knew.

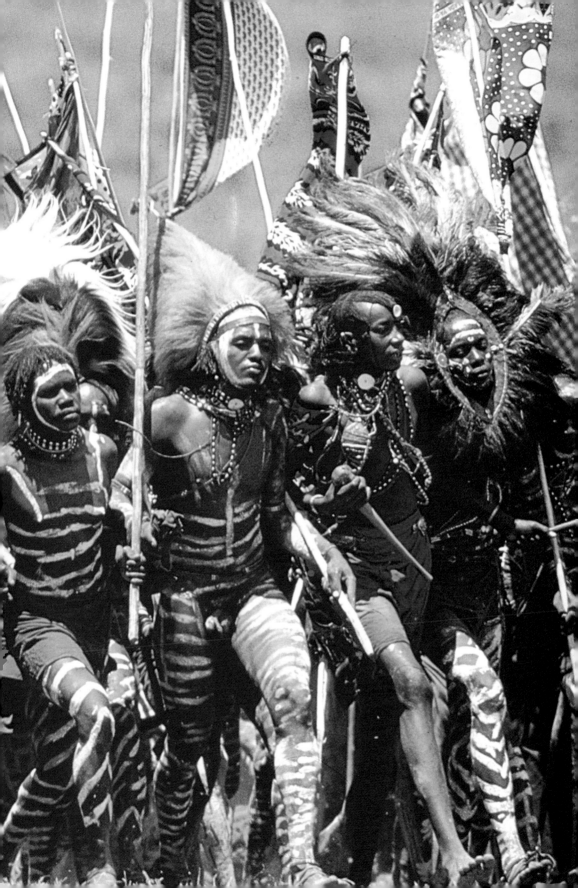

The separation of body from mind

One of the most significant causes of our
estrangement from our bodies is the idea, prevalent in
western society, of mind and body, and body and
soul, as separate entities. We tend to forget that this
dualism is of cultural, not biological origin. In the
East, there is no such division. Body and mind are
traditionally seen as different aspects of one ultimate
reality, and this holistic approach is reflected in their
religious practices, their medical systems, like
acupuncture, as well as in disciplines, such as the
martial arts or yoga, which encompass body, mind,
and spirit, teaching people to live in harmony with
themselves and the world around them.

Here, by contrast, we suffer from an inbuilt
prejudice against the body, tending to think of it as of
secondary importance to the mind. We have become
conditioned to see the body as something to be tamed
and controlled by the mind and have come to regard
identification with the body as an obstacle to spiritual
development. As a result of this ideological split we
have tended to evolve our minds at the expense of our
bodies.

This inner fragmentation is demonstrated by the
way we regard our bodies as possessions. We tend to
think in terms of "having" a body rather than of
"being" a body. But in reality we are one being – our
bodies are ourselves. Our thoughts and feelings, joys
and fears are all mirrored in our bodies.

The educational bias toward the intellect

Nowhere is the dualism of our thinking more evident
than in our schools, where, from a young age, we
spend much of our time sitting quietly while our
minds absorb knowledge. Apart from at primary level
– where the wisdom of educators such as Montessori
and Froebel has left its mark – and in a few
progressive or alternative schools, our education is
woefully one-sided, giving overriding precedence to
intellectual disciplines, and paying far less attention
to the importance of the body, the senses, the role of

"A child who enters school
today faces a twelve- to
twenty-year apprenticeship in
alienation. He learns to
manipulate a world of words
and numbers, but he does not
learn to experience the real
world."
Rudolf Arnheim

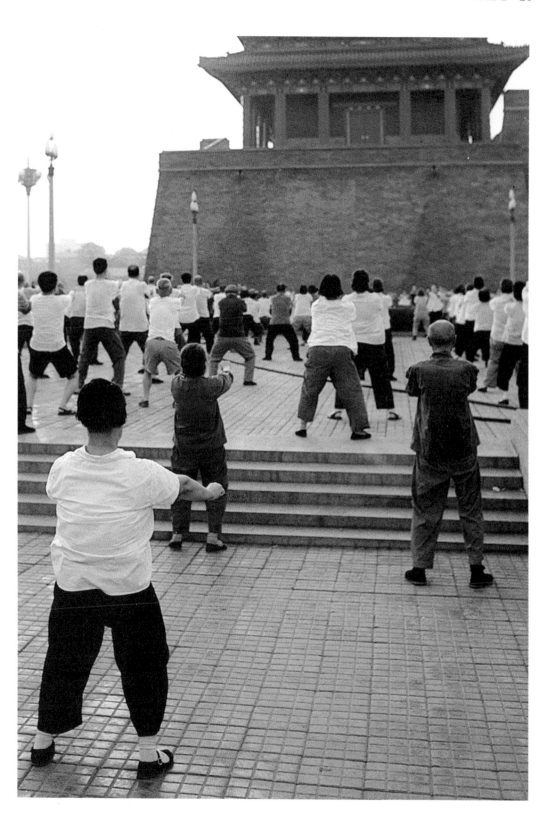

feeling and imagination. At school, we spend countless hours hunched over books, our energy bottled up, using only our heads and our writing hands, while our bodies sit idly waiting – a pattern perpetuated in adult life, if we go on to work in sedentary or desk-bound jobs. We learn that there's a "right" way to sit, to think, to act, to draw and, cowed by the pressure of learning facts, we may begin to lose confidence in our own perceptions and judgements, to lose trust in our own authority. Competitiveness and achievement are encouraged above sharing and co-operation. We are taught to be reasonable and sensible – feeling and emotion tend to be downgraded in favour of logic and reason. "Good" pupils are often those who are most alienated from their own instinctive nature, who learn to toe the line, while "bad" pupils are those whose imagination is strongest, whose type of intelligence falls outside the narrow categories imposed by the schools' curricula. To take account of the whole person and to help us to grow up with a strong sense of self and body awareness, our education needs to be more balanced and holistic, taking into consideration the needs of body, mind, and spirit.

"One of the main difficulties we have to face is that modern education all over the world is chiefly concerned with making us mere technicians...the function of education is not merely to prepare us to pass a few examinations but to help us to understand this whole problem of living – in which is included sex, earning a livelihood, caring for the Earth, being earnest, sharing joy and laughter and yet knowing how to think widely and deeply."
J. Krishnamurti

Learning not to feel

As we grow up, our bodies may also become desensitized and our senses dulled as a means of self-protection, to prevent us from feeling. Theories of child development vary greatly, but most share the view that it is in early childhood that our attitude to ourselves and the world around us is formed – through the experiences we go through, both negative and positive. If our feelings become too difficult to bear, we erect defences in order to survive emotionally, without being overwhelmed. In the view of Wilhelm Reich and his followers, such as Alexander Lowen, these defences become imprinted on our bodies, creating muscle tension and blocking the energy that in health flows freely and

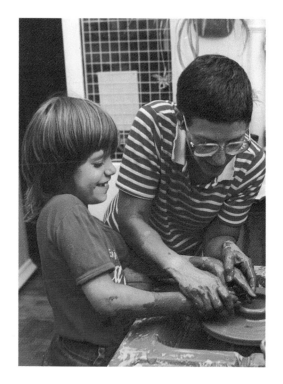

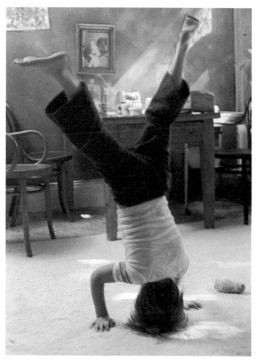

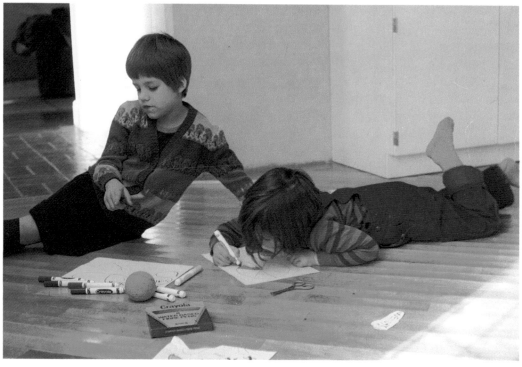

rhythmically, giving us access to our true potential for feeling. This "armouring" may be formed either to deaden our response to hurt or conflict from outside or to suppress "forbidden" or "censored" impulses from inside. But either way, our whole well-being suffers. Our vitality is squandered in tension, our sensitivity and feeling capacity are blunted, and our ability to relate honestly and spontaneously to others is diminished. The armouring creates a network of tension in our muscles and energy blocks in the parts of the body most affected by the childhood conflict or trauma. The kind of situation that causes us to cut off our feelings may not, from an adult point of view, seem that devastating, but the effect on a child that is sensitive can be deep and long-lasting. Thus if as young children we were shamed into suppressing our crying in response to repeated admonishments, such as "don't be a cry-baby" or "big boys don't cry", we get into the habit of tightening our jaws and tensing our diaphragms and chests to hold back the tears. This tightening and suppression can eventually lead to chronic muscular tension, disrupting our breathing pattern and inhibiting our ability to contact and express our feelings freely.

Although learning to become aware of and dissolve the armouring we have built up demands both courage and commitment, the rewards of such work are infinitely worthwhile, for with greater openness and sensitivity comes an increasing capacity for pleasure and for love.

The supremacy of touch

For some, however, loss of body contact appears to come much earlier. In his inspiring book on the significance of the skin, *Touching*, Ashley Montagu underlines the importance of physical contact in early infancy for an individual's total well-being: "Body awareness is produced through stimulation of the body, chiefly through the skin, and this commences at birth, if not before". The first feeling we have of our bodies comes from the loving touch of our parents.

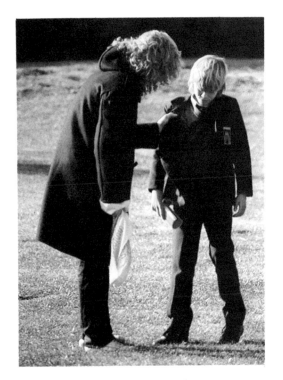

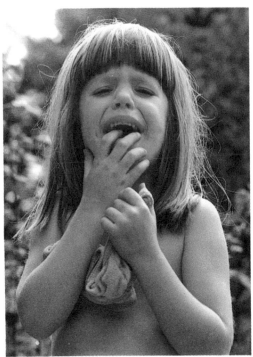

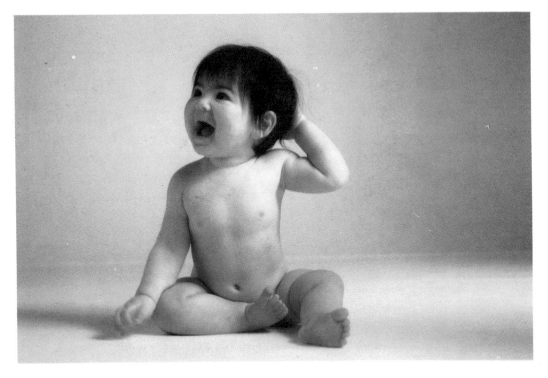

The amount of physical affection we receive in this
pre-verbal period of life, and the ease and pleasure
with which our parents touch us as they feed and bath
us and care for our needs, have a significant influence
on how we feel about ourselves, and on our self-
esteem in later life. Lack of touch in early infancy, by
contrast, is the cause of a whole range of problems in
adult life, both physical and psychological. Babies
who receive insufficient physical contact from their
parents or whose care is interrupted by separation or
illness find it far harder to accept themselves and to
relate intimately to others when they grow up. For we
learn to love through feeling loved ourselves: "The
body-feeling image we have of ourselves as sensitive
or insensitive, sensuous or unfeeling, relaxed or tense,
warm or cold, is largely based on our tactual
experiences in infancy, and subsequently reinforced
by our experiences in childhood" (Ashley Montagu).

*"At the beginning of life, being
stroked, cuddled, and soothed
by touch libidinizes the various
parts of the child's body (and)
helps to build up a healthy
body image and body ego..."*
Anna Freud

In technologically less advanced cultures than our
own, children in general receive far more direct
physical contact. Many infants are carried for the first
couple of years on their parents' bodies and sleep next
to them at night. In some parts of India and Malaya
babies are regularly massaged all over with oil in their
first six months. Among other cultures, such as the
Bushmen of the Kalahari and the Kaingang people of
Brazil, young children receive an immense amount of
physical affection and stimulation.

When they grow up the males of the Kaingang
people often choose to sleep together, not for sexual
purposes, but for the sheer pleasure of the skin
contact.

Parental attitudes and sexuality

Our parents' attitude to their bodies is another
formative factor in determining our sense of our own
bodies, for as children we learn mainly by imitation.
If our parents are at ease with their bodies, if they
move well and express their feelings easily and
spontaneously, then we stand a good chance of
growing up with a positive body image. But if their

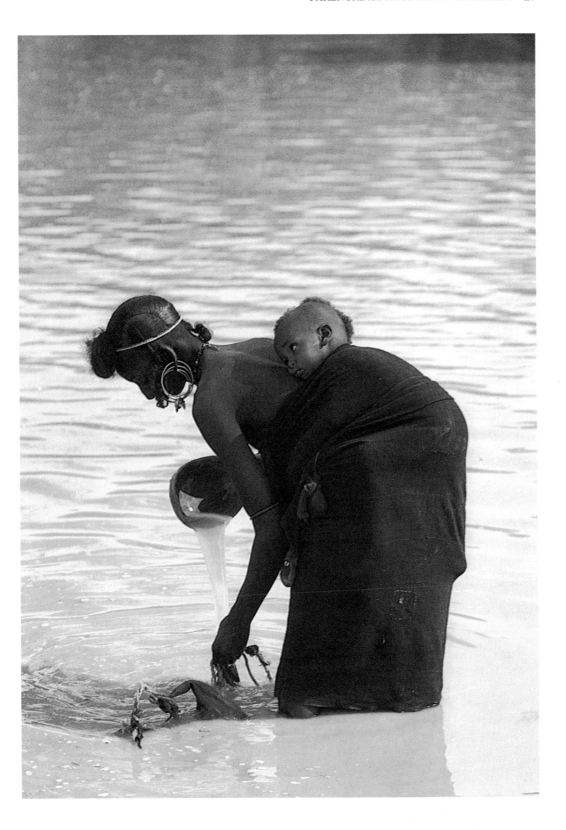

posture and movements are stiff and awkward, their feelings controlled or inhibited, we too are likely to lack confidence in our bodies, to be scared of our feelings and our instinctive drives. Few of us are brought up to love our bodies and to respect and understand their needs.

In their attitudes to sex, parents also have an immense influence on the growing child's body awareness and sensuality, for sexuality is shaped in childhood. In order for children to grow up feeling good about their bodies and their sexual drive, it is vital that they are encouraged to learn about their bodies and body functions in an atmosphere of openness and trust. It is natural for small children to enjoy exploring and playing with their bodies and engaging in infantile sex play with their friends, but all too many parents, through their own inhibitions, are embarrassed by their children's emergent sexuality and unwittingly stifle their curiosity. In families where sex is not talked about freely, children may grow up feeling ambivalent about their bodies and confused or guilty about their "forbidden" feelings, and in consequence find it harder to relate intimately as adults. Even today, despite more widespread sex education in schools, ignorance and inhibition abound. In less "civilized" cultures, such as the Ituri or Mbuti in Africa, by contrast, the onset of puberty is widely celebrated with special rites of passage and, thanks to the sexual openness of their elders, lovemaking is openly discussed with adolescents rather than being shrouded in mystery. Curiosity is encouraged rather than suppressed.

Body image and self-consciousness
Finally, one of the most powerful reasons why many of us desert the comfort and safety of our body homes is when we become self-conscious and begin comparing the way we look with others and measuring ourselves against the ideals of physical desirability perpetrated by the media. From a young age we are continually bombarded with images from

television, cinema, and magazines of the "perfect" way to look. As a result many of us grow up with a negative body image, feeling inadequate and uncomfortable in our bodies – wishing our hair was straighter, curlier, or a different colour, thinking we're too tall, too short, too plump or thin. Both in childhood and puberty, insensitive teasing or repeated criticism of the way we look can also be very damaging, lowering our self-esteem. In adolescence, upset at how our bodies are developing, we may stoop to conceal our height, round our shoulders to hide our breasts, dress in loose clothes to cover up our shape. In swallowing the illusion that there's a "right" way to look, we may cease to regard our bodies as a source of pleasure and adventure and, failing to recognize our uniqueness, reject the way we are. In its most extreme and tragic form, this rejection of our bodies and our sexuality can lead to the "starving" disease, anorexia nervosa.

Reinhabiting the temple

Learning to free the body is not easy. Our defences and inhibitions have become ingrained in our whole way of being from a lifetime of habit, and dissolving our conditioning takes time as well as discipline and commitment. The process of unblocking can be painful and confronting, reawakening old anger, hurts, and fears, and without such strong defences we will naturally feel more vulnerable and sensitive. But the task of becoming more aware of our bodies and ourselves, and reawakening our senses, is infinitely rewarding. As we become aware of our self-limiting armour we can gradually begin to let go of it. We can discover a new sense of unity, strength, and coherence and, by dissolving the barriers that divide us, learn to share ourselves more openly and intimately with partners, family, and friends.

"A body is forsaken when it becomes a source of pain and humiliation instead of pleasure and pride. Under these conditions the person refuses to accept or identify with his body... He may ignore it or he may attempt to transform it into a more desirable object by dieting, weight lifting, etc. However, as long as the body remains an object to the ego, it may fulfil the ego's pride, but it will never provide the joy and satisfaction that the 'alive' body offers."
Alexander Lowen

Elements of awareness

The disciplines and techniques featured in the Solowork and Partnerwork sections of this book are all designed to increase your contact with your body and enhance your self-awareness, enabling you in turn to relate more naturally and confidently to other people. But for the techniques to be effective you need to approach them with the right attitude – to regard them not as techniques or exercises to be accomplished, as techniques that will automatically change your way of being, but as explorations and experiences to work with over a period of time.

When you truly inhabit your body, there is no division between your thoughts, your feelings, and your actions. In such a state of unity and congruence you are totally in tune with yourself – when you speak, your voice and your posture, facial expression and gestures all echo and augment what you are saying. Your whole being supports and reinforces a single statement. Think of a dog clamouring to go for a walk, its eyes and bark and wagging tail all speaking of the same excitement and joy. Or watch a child absorbed in a game, where nothing outside it exists. Without this unity, you remain fragmented and scattered. Your words convey one message, your feelings reveal another and your body, perhaps, a third. Through reconnecting with your body and your feelings, you can learn to discover for yourself a more integrated and spontaneous way of being – a way in which your whole being is united in a common purpose or expression.

In endeavouring to increase your body awareness, your most potent tool is a genuine desire to change. Often we may think we want to change the way we are while unconsciously resisting the idea. To implement change in ourselves, first we may need to become conscious of and explore these hidden resistances. Deep down, many of us don't believe change is really possible. Each of us tends to identify ourselves as a certain kind of person – as someone who is cool, lucid, and unemotional, for example, or as someone who tends to feel clumsy and lack confidence in company. We wear our identities and self-images like a suit of clothes and if we are to change them, we need both a strong desire for a deeper contact with ourselves and a high degree of discipline and self-honesty.

How much you gain from the techniques introduced in the book will be directly related to how far you can allow yourself to relax into sensing and experiencing, how deeply you can get in touch with inhabiting your body. This chapter describes the basic principles you need to understand in order to learn how to expand your body awareness. With these principles firmly in mind, you can approach the exercises and techniques that follow with confidence, and make them really work for you.

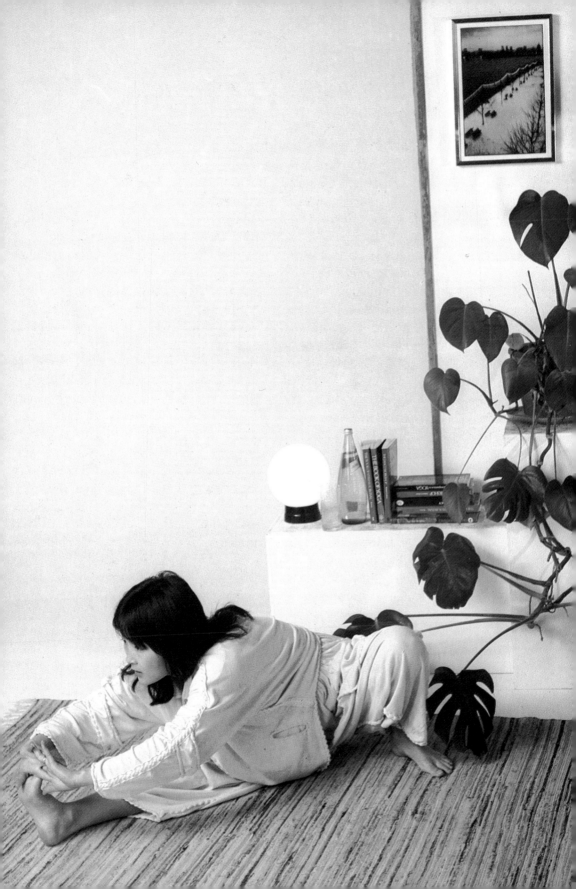

The importance of relaxation

Relaxation is fundamental to inhabiting your body –
if you are tense or wound up, you will not be able to
feel what your body is doing. But the stressful pace of
modern life forces many of us to live out of rhythm
with ourselves and frequently you may find it hard to
let go of the worries and concerns of your daily life
when you come to try out one of the techniques
featured in the book. At such times it's best to spend
five to ten minutes unwinding and relaxing before
you start, to get your attention back into your body.

Take off your shoes and undo or remove any items
of clothing that restrict movement or breathing –
belts, ties, tight buttons, and so forth. Lie down on
the floor (or your bed), with your arms by your sides
and your legs outstretched, a comfortable distance
apart. Close your eyes. Feel your body supported by
the floor, and allow your breathing to become deeper,
until you are inhaling and exhaling slowly and
rhythmically. Now, working systematically up your
body, tense and relax each part in turn. Begin with
your feet. Lift both feet a few inches off the floor...
tense them... hold them there for a moment or two...
then relax and drop them down. Repeat the same
sequence with your legs... your buttocks... your
chest...your hands and arms. Pull your shoulders up
around your ears... hold them there... then relax them
down. Then squeeze your face up tight into a point
around your nose... keep it tense... then allow it to
relax. Breathe in slowly, and as you breathe out feel
your body soften and melt into the floor. In your
mind's eye, visualize yourself in a boat. Feel the gentle
rocking of the boat and listen to the sound of the
water lapping against the sides. Enjoy the warmth of
the sun on your body as you slowly drift downstream.

At the end of this relaxation sequence, open your
eyes and come back to the room gradually. Lie still
for a few moments before slowly getting up.

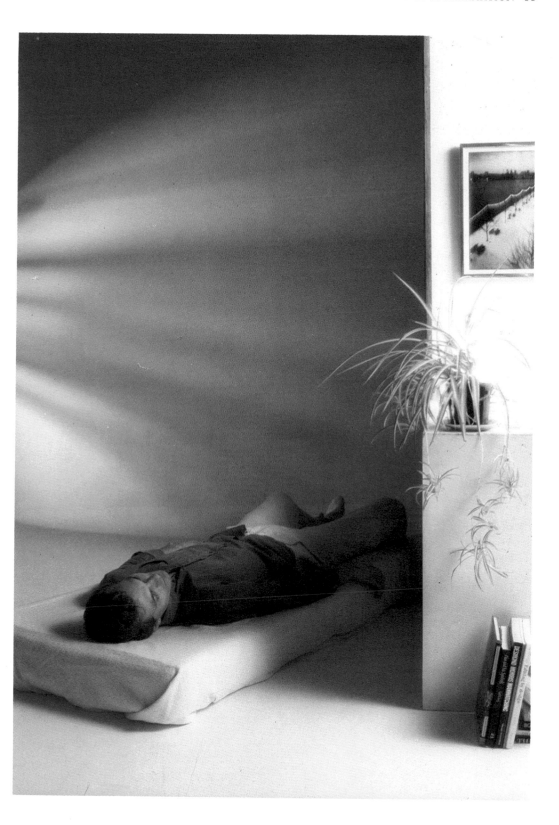

Attitude and the beginner's mind

Cultivating the right attitude to yourself is an
essential part of developing your body awareness. If
you are continually questioning or criticizing yourself
as you try an exercise, for instance, you will block the
feeling of your own experience. You need to put
yourself wholeheartedly into what you are doing, into
the feeling engendered in your body by moving,
standing, sitting, or breathing in a particular way.
Much of the time we tend to operate on "automatic
pilot" when exercising, mindlessly following
instructions. Or else we get hung up on self-
consciousness, on wondering if what we are doing
looks right.

Whether you are doing a breathing exercise,
learning an African dance, or giving your partner a
massage, the aim is to listen to the messages and
sensations that speak from within. If you can get the
feeling right, if you can get a sense of the energy
flowing through your body, you will gain far more
than if you mechanically imitate a technique, joylessly
straining to carry out an instruction or to put your
body into the required position. You need to learn to
follow the dictates of your body rather than leading
yourself with your mind – to let the exercise come to
you, instead of attempting to consciously direct your
experience. Each time you do an exercise, approach it
as if for the first time. Try to develop a "beginner's
mind", coming to every technique openly,
spontaneously, without preconceptions,
expectations, or goals. Be childlike, thinking of each
thing you learn not so much as an exercise to be
accomplished or perfected but as an exploration or
adventure to be experienced. Stay in the fullness of
the moment, trusting your own experience to bring
you what you need.

Awareness and staying present

In learning to reawaken your senses and fully inhabit
your body, another skill you need to develop is a
capacity for sustained awareness or attention. When

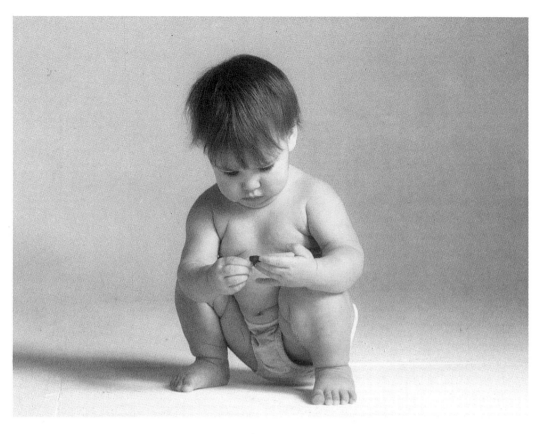

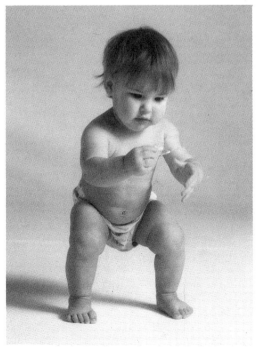
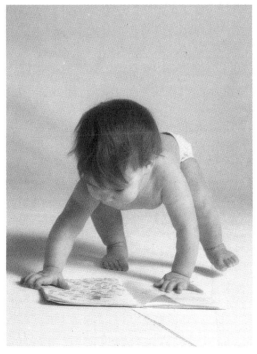

you engage in one of the bodymind disciplines taught
in later chapters, you may find yourself inhibited or
distracted from experiencing your body by a constant
stream of thoughts. This restlessness of the mind
prevents you from staying focused in the present
moment.

In order to be able to perceive and respond to the
sensory messages from your body, you need to train
your awareness, heighten your ability to be fully
present, and learn to quieten your rational mind. The
"rational mind" refers to the thinking, judging,
analysing, computerlike faculty that normally directs
us in our everyday lives. Awareness, or the observing
mind, has a far broader view and a higher
perspective; it comes into being when the rational
mind quietens down.

Quietening the rational mind means watching your
thoughts, without identifying with them. If you
pursue them, you give them more energy, whilst if
you resist them or criticize yourself for being
distracted, you disturb your concentration more. You
need to learn simply to observe them and let them go,
as you would watch clouds drifting across a clear blue
sky and disappearing into the distance. The more you
can lessen the hold of your rational mind, the more
you will be aware of and in touch with the numerous
sensations in your body. And the more you learn to
pay attention to the subtle sensory messages you can
perceive when the mind is quiet, the stronger your
awareness or your observing mind will become. By
training your awareness you can learn to experience
how you stand or move, which parts of your body
you can feel clearly and which are insensitive or cut
off. And once you have recognized your own
individual body map, you can begin to release your
holding patterns and move more freely and sensually.

Emotional release and acceptance
In practising the techniques in this book you are likely
to experience a variety of unfamiliar body sensations
or emotions as you begin to let go of feelings you have

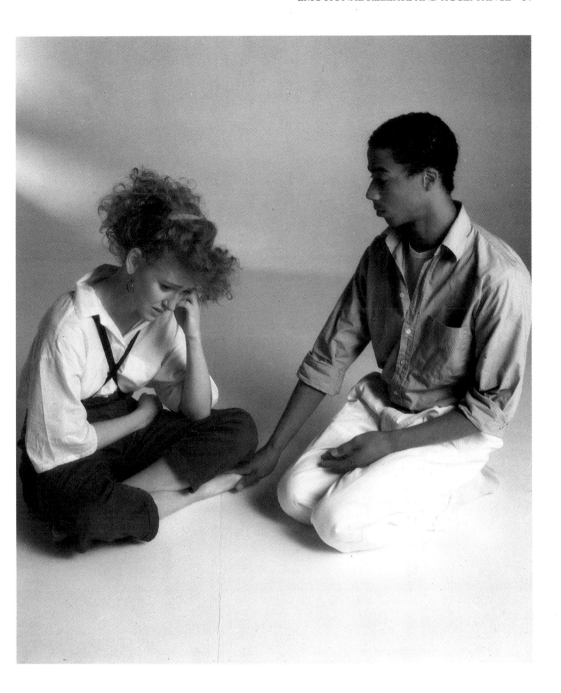

held on to for years – feelings of pain or pleasure, of loneliness, sadness, joy, anger, or fear.

The intensity or suddenness of these feelings may surprise you – at times you may even wonder if the exercises are creating problems that were not there before. In fact, they are merely uncovering layers of feeling that have been suppressed and that up till now have been obstructed or hidden from your awareness by your defences in the form of tension. You should welcome these sensations, for they are a sign that energy is moving, and that you are making a deeper contact with yourself. As you become more sensitive and aware, and allow yourself to live more in the here and now, your capacity for and tolerance of both pleasurable and painful feelings will increase.

Crying or feelings of loneliness or pain are common reactions. If you are on your own, try simply to accept and stay with whatever you are feeling, allowing the tears to flow. Unless you feel overwhelmed, don't resist or tighten against your feelings, nor attempt immediately to regain control. Analysing your experience or trying to work out what originally prompted these feelings will bring you back into your head, out of the reality of the experience. Some of the exercises may also put you in touch with feelings of anger or frustration. You will find some helpful techniques for discharging your anger on pages 166-8.

If you are with your partner while he or she is going through an emotional release, your job is simply to be attentively present. Often we will comfort another for our own peace of mind. It may have taken years for your partner to reach these feelings, and too much comfort can be suppressive. Similarly, don't try to solve your partner's problem or suggest what might help – simply allow him or her to explore and express his or her feelings freely.

SOLOWORK

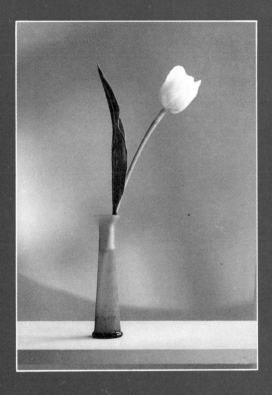

Rediscovering the body
Self-massage

Many of us feel embarrassed by our bodies and unconsciously reject the way we look, wishing to conform to stereotypes of beauty. In some this sense of alienation is profound, resulting in a crippling lack of confidence and trust and in feelings of physical awkwardness and unease. In many more the effect is less extreme, but even those who pride themselves on the way they look are often similarly afflicted once the mask of self-assurance drops.

One of the main problems is that we tend to connect with how we look from the outside rather than with how we feel from the inside. Taken in by the seductive promises of the advertising industry, we seem to think that by making ourselves more presentable outwardly – through buying the right clothes, say, or trimming our bodies to the desired shapes – we will automatically feel better about ourselves inside. But by making us so reliant on outside stimuli, this approach is ultimately self-defeating.

Real inner confidence in the body has little to do with looks or proportions. You can meet people who by any standards are unusually good-looking and yet don't feel it, and others who on the surface are far less attractive and yet possess an ease with themselves and a type of sensuality that is magnetic. Such inner assurance and body awareness stem from self-acceptance and can be gained by learning to acknowledge and appreciate your body.

In this chapter we look at ways to help you befriend your body, through exercises in self-observation and through touch. By practising these techniques, you learn to become aware of and to release tensions and inhibitions about your body, to reclaim parts of yourself you have neglected or cut off from, and to accept yourself as you are.

Your body tells the story of your life and reflects both how you feel and what you think. By gazing at yourself naked in a mirror, you can release the memories and feelings trapped inside, and, in freeing yourself from preconceived ideas, learn to appreciate yourself for your uniqueness and see yourself through new, more compassionate eyes.

Self-massage is a marvellous way of acquainting yourself with your whole body. By bringing your awareness to areas which have felt tense or disconnected, you can help to release the mental and emotional blocks that have been held there, thus restoring these areas to your awareness and expanding your capacity for pleasure. You might find the idea of exploring your body and massaging yourself a little odd at first – taboos about masturbation have left many of us with a vestige of guilt about allowing ourselves to feel pleasure from our own touch. But in fact, by having a better relationship with your own body, you will also enable yourself to give and receive pleasure more freely, enhancing your relationship with your partner.

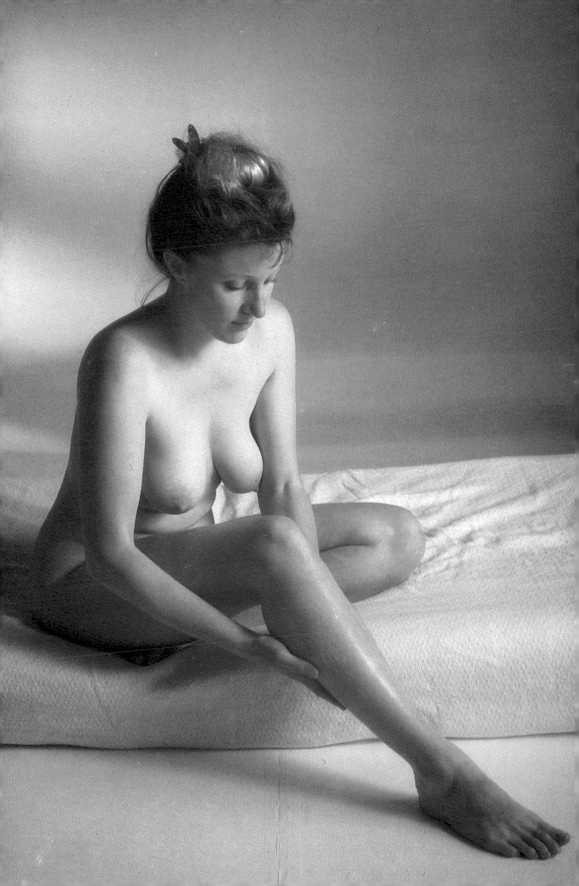

Drawing your inner experience

Your body has an innate intelligence. It contains within itself the answers to many of its own problems. Most of the time, however, the rich inner guidance the body can provide lies beyond your reach. In this exercise, by relaxing and slowing down your thoughts, you make a deeper contact with your body, in order to gain access to the feelings held in a particular part – a part of yourself that causes you pain or embarrassment or a part from which you feel cut off. In this way you can bring inhibitions, tensions, or fears – feelings that are normally hidden from view – from an unconscious to a conscious level, and discover what you can do to resolve them. All you need to do the exercise is a pad of blank paper and some coloured wax crayons or pencils. In the light of what you learn, you may like to massage the part of the body chosen.

Problem and solution
The drawing below was done by a man who chose his head as his problem area.

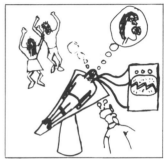

Associated with it were memories of being ill as a child and undergoing many medical tests, at a time when there was a lot of friction between his parents. He also felt that he couldn't express his feelings. His "solution" (below) shows him on top of a hill, receiving the healing energies of the sun and moon.

Sitting comfortably on a chair or on the floor, close your eyes and bring your awareness inside your body.

Feel your buttocks and feet supporting you and, for a few moments, simply watch your breath coming in and going out. Now let your awareness travel to a part of your body that draws your attention. Stay focused in that part and discover how you feel about it...

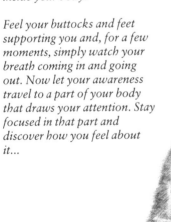

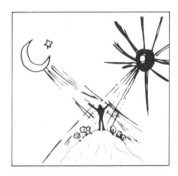

...Now see if any colour, symbol, or memory suggests itself to you linked with the part on which you are focusing. When you feel ready, open your eyes and, taking your paper and colours, draw your experience of your problem area.

When you have finished, take a fresh sheet of paper and draw a solution to your problem.

Mirror-gazing

Most of the time we only stop to look at our reflections to check if we look presentable, to shave, or put on make-up. If we do cast more than a passing glance in the mirror, it is often to criticize ourselves for not living up to our expectations of how we think we should look rather than merely to observe or admire what we see. In this exercise, you simply gaze at yourself naked in a mirror in order to learn to accept yourself and develop the same loving relationship with your own body that you would wish to have with a lover. It's important that you regard yourself compassionately, without judgement, just as you would look at a small child or a close friend. You may find this hard to do initially, however, or get drawn into criticizing aspects of yourself you wish were different. Gazing at your reflection may also awaken memories, or feelings of sadness or loneliness. Simply register whatever thoughts or feelings arise, talking to yourself in the mirror if you like. They are all part of the process of getting to know and love yourself a little better – and it is only by expressing and accepting your feelings that you can begin to make a change.

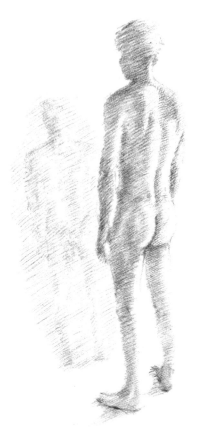

Warm the room, dim the lighting and set aside about 15-30 minutes when you can remain undisturbed. Take off your clothes and any jewellery you are wearing and stand in front of a large mirror, ideally a full-length one.

Start by making eye contact with yourself, then simply allow your gaze to travel slowly down your body, from the top of your head to your feet, letting it rest where it chooses.

Use a hand mirror to look at the back and sides of your body too. If you repeat the exercise periodically, you will find that your perception of yourself gradually changes.

Self-massage

Getting to know and appreciate your body through touch is an important part of self-acceptance, as well as of discovering how to be a good lover. Self-massage will show you which parts of your body you are happy to touch, and which you reject and instinctively shy away from touching. By gently stroking these parts you not only bring energy to them, but can heal the rift caused by cutting them off. Accept it if your touch becomes sexual, but don't get too absorbed. The aim here is to learn to acknowledge your whole body and to extend the boundaries of your capacity for pleasure beyond the most obvious erogenous zones. You can see how effective self-massage can be by spending a few moments simply stroking one of your legs, then lying back, knees up, and comparing how your two legs feel. You will most likely find that the leg you have touched feels lighter and more vibrant. It's good to concentrate on just one part of the body in a session of massage, but from time to time you would also do well to rub some lotion, cream, or oil over your entire body, to give yourself a feeling of wholeness.

Centering

Before beginning a massage, you need to take some time to relax, and bring your awareness into your hands. Kneel or sit comfortably on the floor, or on a chair, hands palms up on your knees or thighs, eyes closed. Now turn your attention to your breath. Just watch it coming in and out, as you might watch waves breaking on a beach. Then begin to focus on your *hara* or lower belly. As you inhale, imagine your breath coming down and filling your belly, and as you exhale, imagine it coming up your torso, down your arms and out of your hands. Continue for a few moments, then slowly raise your hands in front of you and imagine you are holding a ball of light or energy between them. Explore how large the ball is by moving your hands apart and together again. When you are ready, relax your hands in your lap and open your eyes.

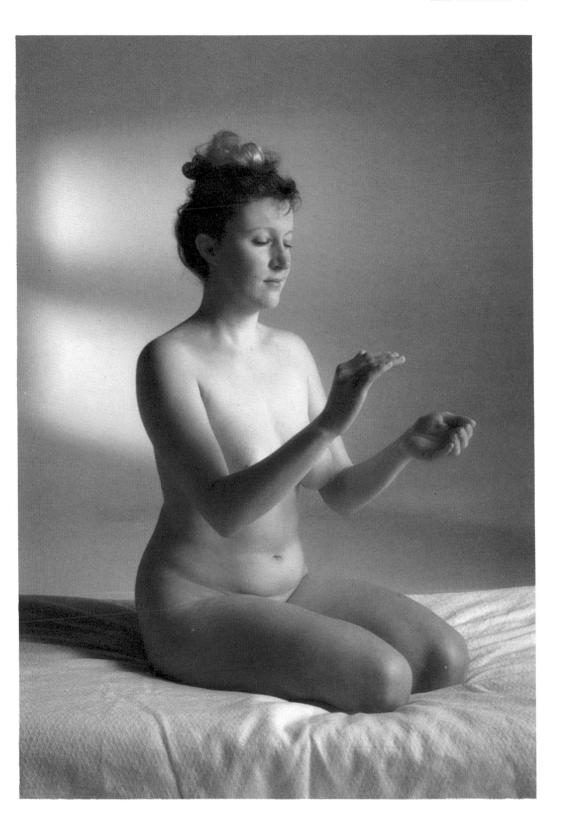

Befriending your body

To enjoy massaging yourself you need to create the right ambience. Warmth, comfort, quiet, and low light are all essential. Find a position that is relaxing and comfortable. Lying on your back or side may be good for some parts, but for others it's easier to sit or kneel down. Have a fragrant body lotion or massage oil ready for use, if you need it. Start by centering yourself, then let your hands settle gently on a part of your body that beckons you. You need have no set route or sequence – sometimes you may feel like spending half an hour on one part, such as the face, at other times you may want to explore the whole body. Be playful and inventive, letting your own sense of pleasure and spirit of discovery dictate where your hands go and how they move. Above all, work slowly and rhythmically, closing your eyes so that you can focus all your attention on sensation.

You may feel like caressing your face with long soothing strokes, like a mother comforting a sleepy child...

...Or you might prefer to work more deeply with your thumbs and fingers around an area of tension, like the jaw muscles or eye sockets. Explore your face thoroughly, as if you were a blind person learning to recognize it for the first time.

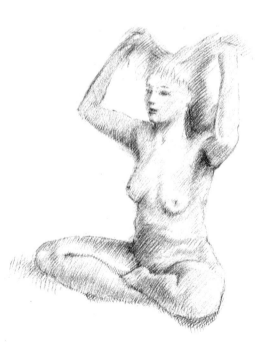

Repeatedly combing your fingers through your hair or gently rubbing your scalp, as if shampooing it, can be immensely relaxing, especially if you tend to live in your head.

See how it feels if you draw your hair out from your scalp, pulling your fingers slowly off the ends, as if to extend the hair.

Bridging the head and the body, the neck often suffers more than its fair share of stress. Yet it receives less attention than most other parts of the body. The easiest way to explore it is to sit with your head bent forward.

See how it feels to stroke both hands firmly up from the base of the neck to the base of the skull, or to draw your hands slowly apart, moving from the neck vertebrae out and around to the front.

As well as being a highly sensitive and erogenous zone, the chest and breast area is also linked to our emotions...

The belly too is a very vulnerable and sensuous area. Go very slowly, working in large circles around your belly, using the whole of your hand. See how it feels to rub in more deeply with your fingers under the ribcage and right down to the pubic bone...

...Bring loving care to your touch, using your hands either singly or together to explore the whole area. And, whether you are male or female, let go of any taboos that may inhibit you from the idea of caressing your own breasts, allowing yourself to enjoy your own touch.

...Try, too, hugging yourself then gradually drawing your forearms and hands apart and off your sides.

Try some long, slow strokes, sweeping down from the top of your arm and off your hand, to give you a sense of your arm as a whole. Stroking repeatedly and very gently down your upper arm, then your lower arm, feels very calming and comforting.

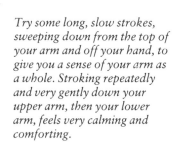

Exploring one of your own hands with the other is an unusual sensation at first, used as we are to shaking or holding hands with others. It also gives you a unique opportunity to see how it feels to give and receive at the same time.

Try working with your thumb into the fleshy areas of the palm, and stretching and squeezing each finger.

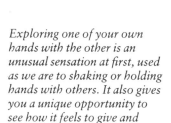

The most comfortable way to reach the whole of your buttocks is by lying on your side. The buttock muscles often hold an amazing amount of tension and it can be surprisingly satisfying to massage them.

Cover the whole area, from the hip joint to the base of your spine. In this position you can also massage your lower back.

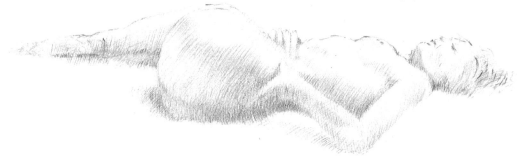

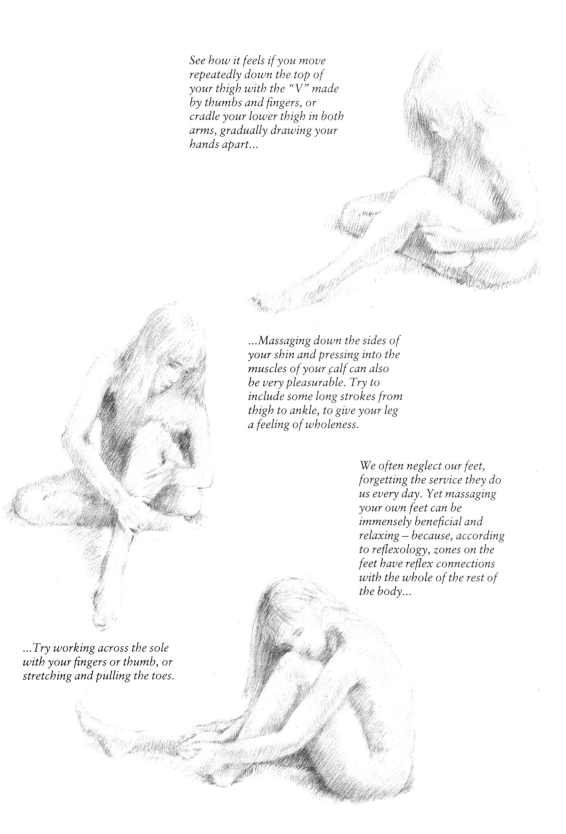

See how it feels if you move
repeatedly down the top of
your thigh with the "V" made
by thumbs and fingers, or
cradle your lower thigh in both
arms, gradually drawing your
hands apart...

...Massaging down the sides of
your shin and pressing into the
muscles of your calf can also
be very pleasurable. Try to
include some long strokes from
thigh to ankle, to give your leg
a feeling of wholeness.

We often neglect our feet,
forgetting the service they do
us every day. Yet massaging
your own feet can be
immensely beneficial and
relaxing – because, according
to reflexology, zones on the
feet have reflex connections
with the whole of the rest of
the body...

...Try working across the sole
with your fingers or thumb, or
stretching and pulling the toes.

Breathing and voicework

The way you breathe reflects the way you live. Breathe well and your health and quality of life are immeasurably enhanced; breathe poorly and both your vitality and your capacity for feeling are impoverished. Breathing is the one body function that can be either voluntary or involuntary, bridging the conscious and the unconscious. By learning to deepen your breathing you can alter the way you are feeling or thinking and discover a new sense of stability and calm. Of all the ways of increasing body awareness, learning to breathe more freely and fully is surely one of the simplest and most effective.

When you breathe freely, the diaphragm, belly, and chest undulate with the rhythm of each breath, and the whole body is energized with life-giving oxygen. Watch a young child or an animal breathe and observe how the body moves when breathing is natural and relaxed. Sadly, as adults most of us have lost this knack and breathe shallowly, without making full use of the diaphragm. Muscular tension is largely to blame for shallow breathing – tension that has evolved over years. Many are taught in childhood to stand up straight, with chest out and belly in, and this "military" posture chronically tightens the breathing muscles. In addition to adopting "bad" postural habits, we may also unconsciously restrict our breathing as a way of suppressing painful emotions, for the depth of our breathing is related to the richness and intensity of our feelings. As we grow up many of us learn to control rather than express our deepest feelings, and this inevitably means tightening our breathing muscles and tensing our chests or bellies, the seat of our feelings. In the process of distancing ourselves from feelings of sadness, anger, or fear, however, we also block the free flow of energy in the body and diminish our capacity for pleasure.

In restricting our breathing, our voices suffer too – for if the throat, diaphragm, and belly are tight or tense, the strength and resonance of the voice are naturally affected. Learning to deepen our breathing and release the patterns of holding in our bodies will also help to open up our voices.

The exercises in this chapter will help you to free both your breathing and your voice, by making you aware of the tensions in your body that inhibit natural breathing, and teaching you how to extend your breathing capacity. But for these exercises to make a real difference it's a good idea to monitor your breathing while you go about your daily life. From time to time, just observe your breath and you will begin to see that thoughts or feelings can disrupt your natural rhythm and make you hold your breath. Don't force yourself to breathe differently, however. The aim is not to impose a new pattern of controlled breathing but to allow you gently to rediscover your own natural rhythm.

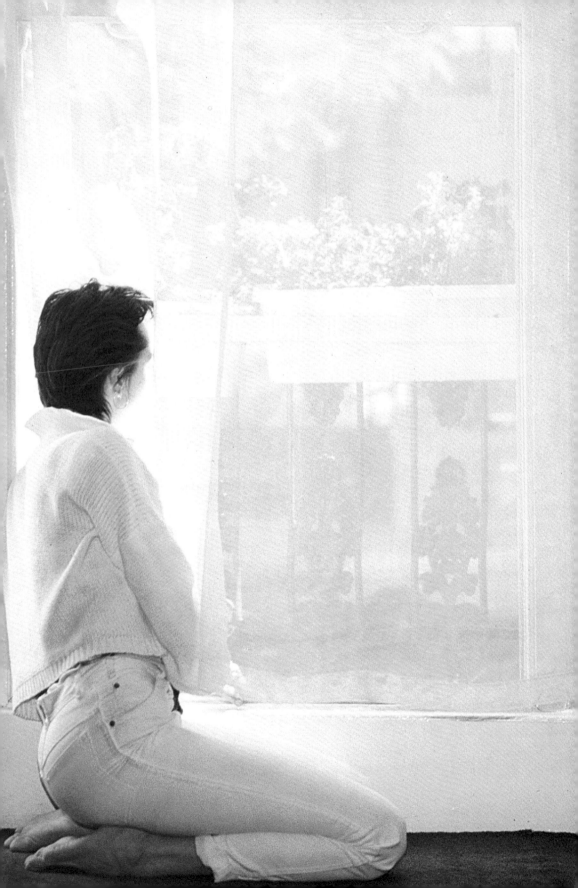

How do you breathe?

Your breathing changes according to what you are doing – when you are active, it tends to be faster and shallower, while when sleeping or relaxing it changes to a slower, deeper rhythm. Many of us, however, don't use our full breathing capacity and breathe shallowly and unevenly as a general rule, depriving ourselves of the relaxation and calm that naturally accompany deep abdominal breathing. To breathe freely, your belly should be relaxed, your back straight, and your shoulders down, not hunched. In addition, your diaphragm, the dome-shaped sheet of muscle that separates the lungs from the abdominal organs, needs to be flexible. When the diaphragm is tight, your breathing capacity is restricted and your feelings and energy are blocked. Many people make the mistake of pulling in their bellies or raising their shoulders when they inhale, instead of allowing the belly, followed by the chest, to expand. When practising any of the breathing exercises that follow, pay attention to making a full exhalation, ridding your lungs of all the stale air, and allow the inhalation to follow spontaneously.

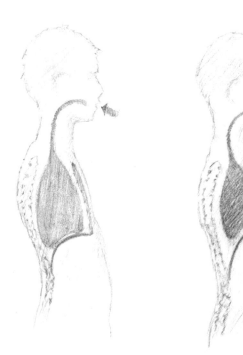

The anatomy of breathing
In a normal full breath, the diaphragm contracts and moves down when you breathe in, pushing the belly out and pushing the ribs up and outward. This expansion of the chest creates a vacuum so that air is sucked in to the lungs. When you exhale, the diaphragm moves up and the ribcage and abdomen contract, expelling air from the lungs.

Finding your diaphragm

In order to improve your breathing, you first need to become aware of your present breathing pattern. This exercise will show you how freely your chest and belly move when you breathe and bring you in touch with the motion of the diaphragm. It will also help to expand your breathing capacity, by stretching the breathing muscles and diaphragm.

Lie down on your back and try breathing into your belly only, feeling it rise and fall, without moving your chest. Put your hands on your chest to check that it remains still. Continue breathing like this for a few minutes.

Next breathe only into your chest, feeling it swell and subside, and place your hands on your belly this time, to see that it does not move.

Which did you find easiest? Do you tend to be a chest breather or a belly breather? Now put your arms down by your sides and exhale. With your breath out, bear down, puffing out your belly, then release. Repeat this several times until you need to take another breath.

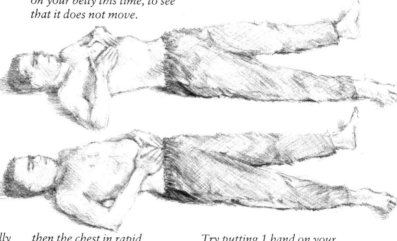

After trying this for a few moments, reverse the movement, sucking your belly in and puffing out your chest after an exhalation. As before, repeat the in/out movement then relax, breathing normally. Finally, combine the last 2 movements. After exhaling, alternately puff out the belly

then the chest in rapid succession. You can feel your diaphragm moving just under your ribs. Relax for a little while then repeat, this time pumping faster. Notice how your breathing feels now, after completing the whole exercise.

Try putting 1 hand on your belly and 1 on your chest and feel how the belly, then the chest, swells as you inhale and subsides, in reverse order, as you exhale.

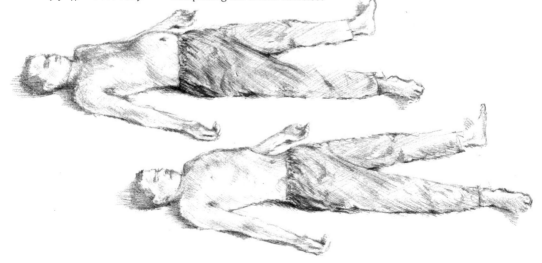

The Jellyfish

Pulsation – the rhythmic movement of expansion and contraction – is common to all living things, from the most primitive life forms upward. In the human body, it underlies many functions, from the rhythmic pumping of the heart to the ebb and flow of the craniosacral rhythm. But it is in breathing that we link ourselves most closely with the pulsation of life at a feeling level. The Jellyfish is a three-part exercise that combines rhythmic body movements with the natural pulsation of breathing, contracting or drawing the body in toward the centre with every exhalation and expanding it outward with each inhalation. In the beginning, you may find you need to synchronize your breathing with your leg movements consciously, but in time your own natural rhythm will develop by itself, allowing you to enjoy the oceanic feeling of the pulsation. Performing the exercise should be pleasurable, for it increases the flow of energy in the body, but this can make you feel a little anxious if you are not used to it. Take it one step at a time, waiting until you feel happy with part one before moving on to the next.

The Jellyfish
1. Lie down on the floor, arms out to the sides. Bend your knees and put your feet down, parallel to one another, about 6 inches apart. Breathe in, then, as you breathe out, bring your knees up toward your body, wrapping your hands around them to press them in to your chest. As you breathe in again, bring your arms out to the sides and lower your knees (your feet need not touch the floor). Continue for about 5 minutes, developing your own natural rhythm.

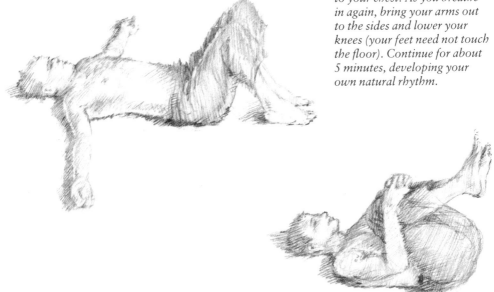

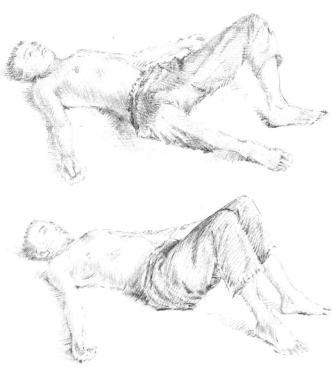

2. Begin as before, with feet flat, and arms out to the sides. But this time, as you breathe in, allow your knees to fall out to the sides and your feet to rotate a little; as you breathe out, bring your knees together again, until they are close but not touching. Open your legs only as wide as is comfortable – don't strain. As you repeat this pattern, try to make the movement smooth and flowing, continuing for 5 minutes.

3. Repeat the same pattern as in part 2 of the exercise, but now include your pelvis in the movement. As you breathe in, dropping your knees out to the sides, tilt the pelvis down, very slightly, pressing the base of your spine against the floor; as you breathe out, bringing your knees together, tilt the pelvis up slightly, lifting the base of the spine off the floor.

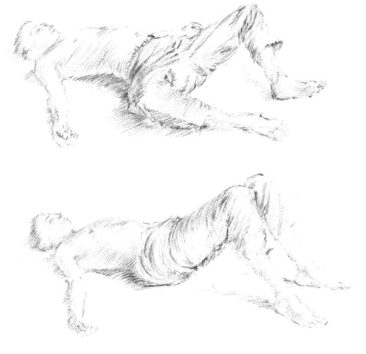

Alternate nostril breathing

In the spiritual traditions of many eastern cultures, breath is believed not only to contain oxygen but also to carry the life force or vital energy, known as *prana*, *chi*, or *ki*. In yoga, *pranayama* or the regulation of *prana* through breathing exercises is one of the principal daily practices. *Pranayama* not only energizes the whole body, it also creates emotional stability, and great clarity of mind. Alternate nostril breathing is both soothing and calming, producing a unique sensation of balance between the left and right sides of the body. It is often used prior to meditation as a way of bringing you into the present and stilling the restlessness of the mind. Try to keep your body still and your right shoulder relaxed, not raised, while you practise.

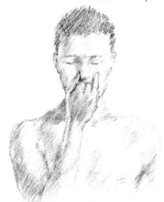

Sit comfortably, cross-legged on the floor or on an upright chair, back straight. Raise your right hand and lower the index and middle fingers into your palm, leaving the thumb and last 2 fingers free (see right). You will use the thumb to close your right nostril, your fingers to close the left.

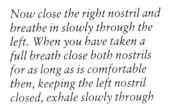

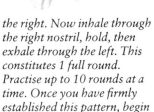

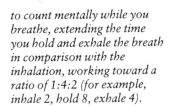

Now close the right nostril and breathe in slowly through the left. When you have taken a full breath close both nostrils for as long as is comfortable then, keeping the left nostril closed, exhale slowly through

the right. Now inhale through the right nostril, hold, then exhale through the left. This constitutes 1 full round. Practise up to 10 rounds at a time. Once you have firmly established this pattern, begin

to count mentally while you breathe, extending the time you hold and exhale the breath in comparison with the inhalation, working toward a ratio of 1:4:2 (for example, inhale 2, hold 8, exhale 4).

Chakra *breathing*

The *chakras* are energy centres that connect the physical body with the subtle body or aura surrounding it. Most traditions recognize seven main *chakras*, ranging up from the base of the spine to the top of the head. Each one relates to a different part of the body as well as to a different function. So in breathing in to a *chakra* you not only energize that centre but also make contact with a realm of behaviour and feeling. In this exercise you focus on four of the *chakras* in turn: the throat *chakra*, associated with self-expression and creativity; the heart *chakra*, related to compassion and unconditional love; the solar plexus *chakra*, associated with emotion, fear, and more personal love; and the *hara*, the *chakra* related to sexuality, vitality and physical power. The exercise ends with breathing in to the genitals and out down the legs, allowing you to ground yourself with your breath.

This breathing technique can also be beneficial if you feel tense or stiff or have a pain. Simply breathe in to the area of pain, then imagine the tension or pain releasing or dissolving as you exhale.

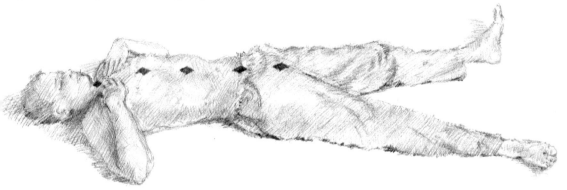

Lie down on your back and relax. Feel your body making contact with the floor. Each time you inhale, you imagine you are breathing in to part of the body, sending your energy to that area. You spend a few minutes focusing your breath on each part in turn. First, rest your fingertips lightly on the throat chakra, *in the little*

hollow above the collarbone, as shown below, and breathe in to that area... Next move your hands to the heart chakra, *in the centre of your chest, and focus your breathing there...*

Then move down to the solar plexus chakra, *just below the breastbone... From there shift your hands to the* hara, *3*

fingerwidths below the navel. Notice any differences in the quality of feeling or thought at each chakra *you come to... Finally, put your hands lightly on your genitals and visualize breathing in to them and out down your legs and feet, so that you end up by grounding yourself with your breath.*

Using the voice

Few of us know the full strength and expressiveness of our own voices. Rigid notions about the "correct" way to speak or sing have robbed many in our culture of a spontaneous delight in exploring the range, beauty, and power of the voice. But throughout most of human history children have learnt to express themselves through chanting and singing as readily as they learn to talk and there are still many parts of the world where everyday activities are accompanied by singing or chanting. Using the full range of the expressive voice enhances our whole well-being.

To project our voices beyond that of normal speech – be it for acting, public speaking, singing, or for our own enjoyment – requires us to use our whole bodies, especially our lungs and vocal equipment, in a way that paradoxically blends relaxation and energy. But finding this balance, and learning to allow the sounds to come through unblocked and resonant, can create an immense reservoir of energy. Far from draining or straining the voice, it becomes possible to use it freely and powerfully, for hours. The instructions that follow will help you to reverse common inhibitions and reclaim your natural voice.

"The voice is the muscle of the soul."
Alfred Wolfsohn
Papers of the Roy Hart Theatre

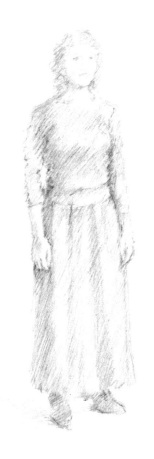

Stance for giving voice
Stand with your feet apart, and feel your connection to the ground. Imagine you are like a tree, with roots extending into the earth. Make sure your knees are not held stiffly back, but have a sense of bounce and flexibility. You'll notice how this gives you a sense of your weight being centered in your pelvis, which also then becomes flexible. This makes it possible to sway gently or move as you give voice, however small the movement, rather than standing stock still, *which stiffens the expressive voice as it does the body. Your shoulders, neck, and jaw should be relaxed but not slouched.*

Positions of head and neck
Imagine that there is a string coming from the crown of your head, gently lifting it, so that your neck and windpipe feel free and open. Without stiffening your neck and shoulders, make sure that your head isn't tilted forward or back.

Opening your mouth

To project your voice most easily and freely, you need to be able to open your mouth wide. First allow your jaw to drop as far as it will without strain. Then form the shape of your mouth into a slight smile, which will lift your upper lip to show your top teeth and slightly lift the corners of your mouth.

Feeling your throat wide open

Whenever you project your voice, you need to have your throat wide open and relaxed. Close your eyes, and with your mouth open, as described above, draw in breath evenly. While experiencing this sensation, imagine some picture that helps you to capture and sustain it. The aim of this is to visualize your throat as a wide open channel, allowing sound through. Common helpful images chosen include a tunnel or cavern mouth. Rather than just breathing out, now try calling with the sound "hey" (without emphasizing the "h"). There is no need to force out breath to make a strong sound. In fact, you can sing or speak loud and clear holding a mirror 3 inches from your mouth, without it misting up.

Experiment with yawning (making sure not to tilt your head back), and you'll notice that the first part of a yawn puts your mouth into an identical shape to this.

Jaw relaxation

To maximize the quality of your voice using the resonance cavities of your face and head, your jaw needs to be loose and relaxed. Keeping your head still, move your lower jaw around into as many shapes and positions as you can without strain, to reduce the tensions that so many of us carry there. Massaging your jaw muscles will also help.

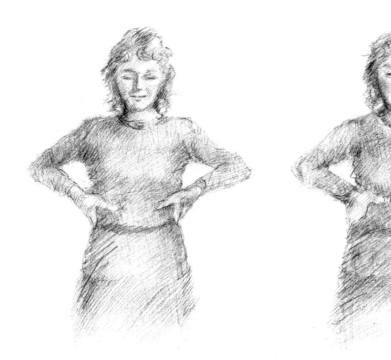

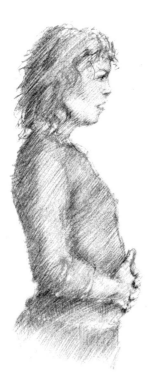

Breathing for giving voice

The kind of inhalation appropriate to support and sustain giving voice requires the main expansion to be in the area of the lower ribs – the lower part of the lungs – which automatically involves the diaphragm. Puffing up the upper chest when you inhale will lead to tension in the shoulders and neck.

As well as expanding your ribcage in the front, you need to feel yourself expanding at the side and back – in fact, in all directions. To help check you're doing this, place your hands on your ribs, as shown above. As you breathe in, see if you can push your hands backward and sideways with the intake of breath.

Energy for giving voice

Place your hands on the front of your abdomen, just above your navel. As you breathe in, this area will of course be part of the expansion. Now, opening your mouth (as described on p.59), give a strong clear call. You will get the best tone when you feel a slight dynamic tension in the muscles under your hand for the duration of the sound. If you allow these muscles to sag, the sound will lose its quality and sustaining power and, in singing, will often drift flat.

Gentle rhythmic movements
Many people find it much easier to free their voices when moving. It helps to release tension, and allows you to relax and "tune in" to the body. After all, throughout history, most chanting and singing have been accompanied by movement – be it work, dance, ritual, or simply walking. Try a rhythmical rocking or swinging movement so that your weight moves forward and back, knees bending gently and arms swinging in co-ordination. Experiment with open vowel sounds that work with the rhythm of the movement.

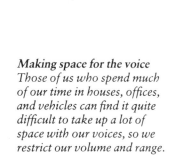

Making space for the voice
Those of us who spend much of our time in houses, offices, and vehicles can find it quite difficult to take up a lot of space with our voices, so we restrict our volume and range.

Imagine yourself on a hillside, on a sunny day, calling in the cows or hollering across a valley where there's an echo. Play with the sounds, enjoying the inner expansion from your breathing, and the sense of filling the space outside.

Grounding

As its name suggests, grounding relates to our connection with the ground and, in a broader sense, to our whole contact with reality. It is associated with all levels of our being – physical, mental, emotional, and spiritual. Being grounded suggests stability, security, independence, having a solid foundation, living in the present rather than escaping into dreams. It means having a mature sense of responsibility for ourselves, "standing on our own two feet", and "knowing where we stand".

Much of our sense of grounding comes from the way we identify with the lower half of our bodies – our feet, legs, pelvis, and belly, the parts of our being concerned with the less conscious, more instinctive functions of movement, digestion, sex, conception, and birth. But as two-legged beings, many of us have become distanced from our biological roots, resulting in a feeling of living up in the air, of being rootless or spaced out. Lacking grounding, we tend to resist the pull of gravity with our bodies, tensing our muscles to stand upright, rather than trusting the earth to hold us up and allowing our weight to be carried by our feet. But grounding is essential if we are to be fully in touch with our bodies, to trust and enjoy our feelings, and to give and receive pleasure freely.

Many of the disciplines in this book will help to increase your groundedness – the chapters on T'ai chi, African dance,

Running, Aikido, and Breathing are especially relevant. Learning to breathe into the belly is vital for grounding, for if your breath is shallow, your contact with reality and with your feelings will be limited. Massaging the lower part of your body is also a good way of improving your grounding.

This chapter contains exercises specifically designed to enhance grounding, some of which derive from bioenergetics. This system, aimed at relaxing physical and emotional blocks, and mobilizing your energy, was developed by Alexander Lowen, and is now widely taught. Many bioenergetic exercises involve putting the body into positions of slight stress to increase the energetic charge, inducing vibrations or streaming sensations through the body. Some may feel a little painful at first or lead to the release of suppressed feelings. But you will find that as the tension in your body dissolves, performing the exercises will become increasingly enjoyable. Practised regularly, they can put you more in touch with your body, and increase your tolerance for pleasure, allowing you to feel more vibrantly alive. Unless otherwise instructed, do the exercises with your eyes open – as infants it is primarily with our eyes that we first make contact with reality. Shutting your eyes can be a way of escaping into a dream world and cutting off your feelings.

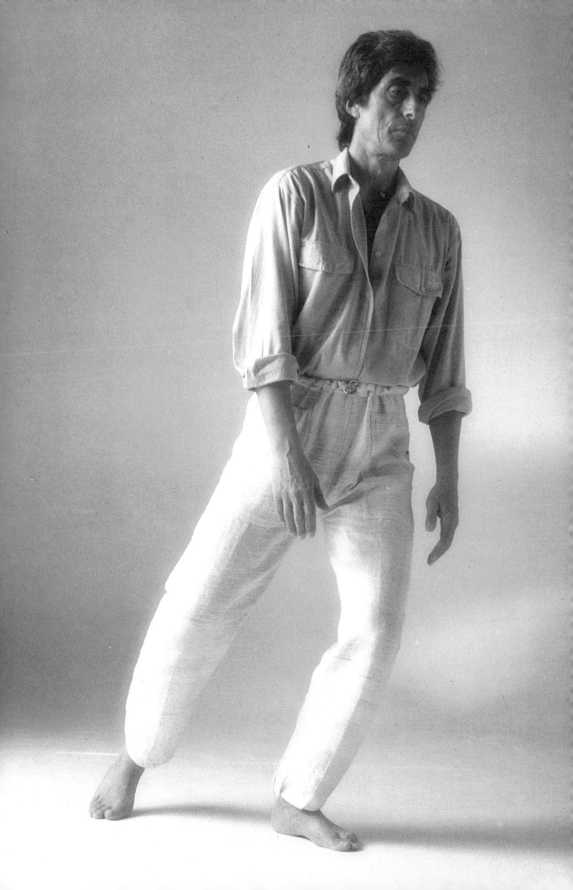

How grounded are you?

The exercises that follow have been chosen to help to improve your grounding, working specifically on loosening energy blocks in particular parts of the lower body, so that your energy can flow more freely. Energy blocks are generally shown in muscle tensions and inflexibility, causing parts on either side of the block to be pale, cold, and toneless or by contrast more highly charged and muscle-bound. Incorporating the whole of the lower body, the two exercises described here will help you to distinguish where your own particular tensions and blocks are located, enabling you to target more precisely the parts you need to spend time on. You may find it hard to keep your attention focused in the Grounding Awareness exercise to begin with, but if you persevere, it can provide not only a means of discovering which parts of you are cut off, but also a powerful way of making you feel more grounded.

Grounding awareness
Stand with your legs apart, weight evenly balanced. Bring your awareness to your sacrum at the base of the spine. Now move your awareness slowly down your right leg until, when it reaches your right sole, all your weight is on your right foot. Keep your left foot on the ground. With your weight still on your right foot, move your awareness slowly across to your left sole. Then, as you travel up your left leg, gradually transfer your weight to your left foot so that by the time you reach the sacrum, all your weight is there. Repeat 2-3 times, ending by distributing your weight evenly between both feet.

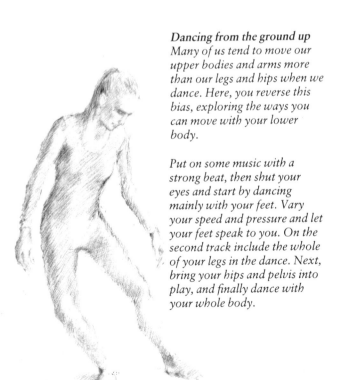

Dancing from the ground up
Many of us tend to move our upper bodies and arms more than our legs and hips when we dance. Here, you reverse this bias, exploring the ways you can move with your lower body.

Put on some music with a strong beat, then shut your eyes and start by dancing mainly with your feet. Vary your speed and pressure and let your feet speak to you. On the second track include the whole of your legs in the dance. Next, bring your hips and pelvis into play, and finally dance with your whole body.

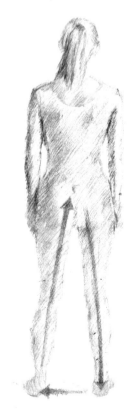

Feet and ankles

Our feet represent our contact with the world around us. Carrying our full weight, they exchange energy with the earth, like the roots of a tree, endowing us with a feeling of connectedness with the ground. But many of us have lost touch with our feet and with them our rootedness, weakening both our sense of balance and our contact with reality. People with suppler, more relaxed feet generally have a more flexible approach to life, while stiff, lifeless feet suggest an inflexible attitude, and collapsed, flaccid feet often accompany insecurity and passivity. Tension in the ankle joints also interferes with our contact with the ground, cutting down the flow of energy between feet and legs. The exercises below help to loosen feet and ankles but, in addition, you can do a lot to assist your groundedness by spending as much time as possible barefoot, and avoiding shoes that squeeze your feet.

Standing and rocking
Stand barefoot, feet apart. Bend your knees and relax, breathing deeply. Now simply rock your weight back and forth from toes to heels. Notice where you put most of your weight – on your right foot or left, the inside or outside of your feet. Rock from side to side too. Then close your eyes and imagine you are standing on warm sand. Imagine roots growing down from your feet, and feel one strong root extending deep into the earth from your coccyx. Feel any tension draining down into the ground.

Repeated weekly, this can change how you stand and walk.

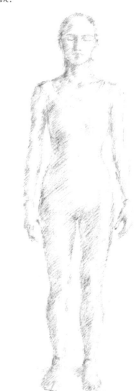

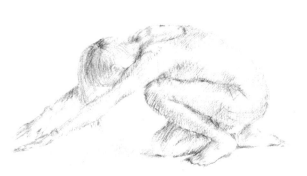

Loosening the ankles
This bioenergetic exercise helps to unblock energy held in the ankles, stretching the Achilles tendons. Kneel down, then raise your left knee and place the foot down flat a few inches behind your right knee. Now shift your weight on to the ball of your left foot, stretch your arms forward, and rock back and forth, pressing your foot into the floor as you rock forward. Try to keep your breathing rhythmical, and the rest of your body relaxed. Repeat, reversing the position of your legs. Kneeling down and sitting back on your heels, spine straight, will also help to loosen your ankles.*

Knees and legs

Among the most common ways of symbolically holding back from life is standing or walking with your knees locked or braced. Learning to stand and move with your knees slightly flexed at all times is one of the most effective principles you can observe in endeavouring to become more grounded. If your legs are either too flaccid or too tense, they will lack feeling, and energy is unlikely to be able to flow fluently through them. Weak, underdeveloped legs often signify a tentative, dependent attitude and an inability to stand up for yourself. Tense, muscle-bound legs suggest a clinging to structure, and a fear of letting go or being spontaneous. Shaking and kicking out (below) are good ways of discovering where the tension lies in your legs. By noticing how hard it is to make them floppy, you will see where and how much you are holding on. The other exercises that follow are bioenergetic; practised consistently, they will enable you to release muscular tension and experience far more sensation in your legs.

"There are two commandments that, if observed, help you become and stay grounded. The first is to keep your knees slightly flexed at all times... The second commandment is to let the belly out."
Alexander Lowen

Kicking out
You can also shake tension out of your legs, especially your knees, by standing as before, keeping your supporting leg slightly bent, then kicking out repeatedly with one leg, letting your heel direct the movement.

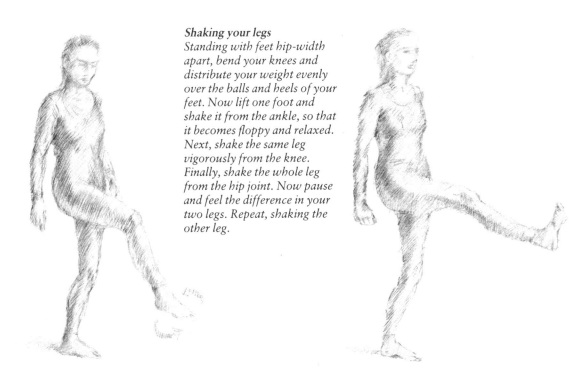

Shaking your legs
Standing with feet hip-width apart, bend your knees and distribute your weight evenly over the balls and heels of your feet. Now lift one foot and shake it from the ankle, so that it becomes floppy and relaxed. Next, shake the same leg vigorously from the knee. Finally, shake the whole leg from the hip joint. Now pause and feel the difference in your two legs. Repeat, shaking the other leg.

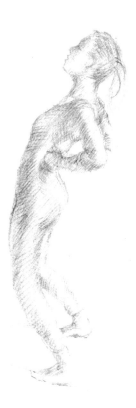

The Bow

Stand with your legs wide apart, toes turned inward, knees slightly bent. Put your fists in the small of your back, just below the waist, and arch back. Let your belly out as far as possible and breathe deeply through your mouth. Your weight should be centered on the balls of your feet and your hips neither tilted forward nor back, so that your body forms a continuous arch shape. When vibrations start to occur in your legs, allow them to happen and surrender to the flow of energy, giving voice to any feelings that come up. Always end by reversing the stretch on your back and discharging the energy built up in your legs by hanging forward, as shown below. If you feel any pain in your lower back after the exercises, lie down, bring your knees up to your chest and clasp your hands around them, then rock back and forth or from side to side.

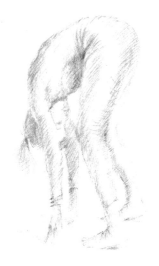

Forward bend

Standing with your feet shoulder-width apart, toes pointing slightly inward, knees slightly flexed, bend forward. Let your head drop down, and touch the floor with your fingertips, but don't put any weight on your hands. Breathe deeply through your mouth into your belly. Thrust your weight forward on to the balls of your feet. Feel your connection with the ground. After a while, your legs will probably start vibrating. If they don't, increase the stretch on the back of your legs by slowly straightening your knees a little. Hold this pose for a minute or 2, allowing yourself to go with the vibrations and to release any feelings triggered by the exercise. Then slowly stand up straight and relax, breathing freely.

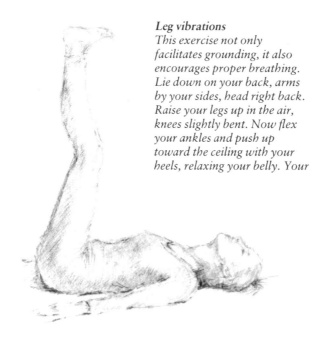

Leg vibrations

This exercise not only facilitates grounding, it also encourages proper breathing. Lie down on your back, arms by your sides, head right back. Raise your legs up in the air, knees slightly bent. Now flex your ankles and push up toward the ceiling with your heels, relaxing your belly. Your legs should start vibrating. If they don't, you can help to prompt the vibrations by bending and straightening your legs. Keep your heels thrust up as your legs vibrate, and breathe easily. Continue for a minute.

As a slight variation, you can use the same starting position to loosen your ankles. Move your feet up and down several times then rotate them, making circles in both directions.

Working on the inner thighs

Tightness in the thighs can inhibit full sexual expression and restrict mobility. This bioenergetic exercise stretches and relaxes the inner thighs, causing waves of pleasurable vibrations in the thighs and pelvic floor. The vibrations also help to deepen your breathing.

Lie down on your back, arms by your sides and head back. Bend your knees, and put your feet about 18 inches apart. Keeping your feet flat on the floor, slowly move your knees as far apart as possible, then slowly move them toward one another until they meet. Keep breathing easily while you move your legs in and out and release any holding in the anus. Continue the movement when the vibrations start to occur.

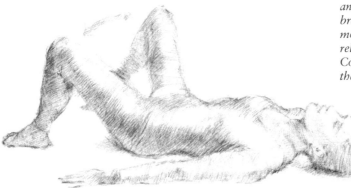

Pelvis and belly

In the East, most notably in the tradition of the martial arts, the *hara* or lower belly is seen as the centre of gravity and the seat of vitality; to be grounded you need to be centered there, rather than higher up the body. Grounding is also closely linked to sexuality – if you are not grounded, you won't be able to give free rein to sexual feelings. In order to enjoy your sexuality with your whole being, you need to be fully in touch with your own instinctual drives and be able to accept and release the charge of sexual energy in your body. Many people, however, unconsciously inhibit or deaden their sexuality by their postures. The belly is pulled in, preventing proper breathing and so restricting sexual feeling in the pelvic area. The pelvis is held permanently tucked forward or cocked back. And the buttocks are tightened, pulling up the pelvic floor, expressing a fear of letting go. To make the most of your sexuality, you need to relax the buttocks, pelvic floor, and anus, release tension from the legs, and restore full mobility to the pelvis.

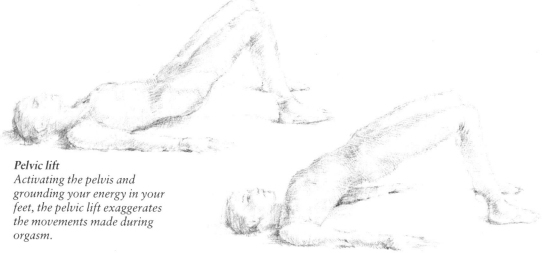

Pelvic lift
Activating the pelvis and grounding your energy in your feet, the pelvic lift exaggerates the movements made during orgasm.

Lie down, bend your knees, and place your feet flat on the floor, about 18 inches apart. Now, very slowly, push down with your feet and begin to lift your pelvis up, then your back, vertebra by vertebra, moving sinuously like a snake, until you are supported only by your head, shoulders, and feet. Take a few deep breaths in this arched position, then come down again equally slowly, keeping your pelvis forward until it rests on the floor. Repeat this movement 5-10 times, enjoying the feeling of energy streaming through your body.

Pelvic rocking

Lie flat on the floor, knees bent, feet hip-width apart. Now slowly move your pelvis back and forth, alternately pressing your sacrum against the floor, then curling it up off the floor, like a dog with its tail between its legs. Synchronize your breathing with this movement, inhaling when you *tilt the pelvis back, exhaling when you tilt it forward. Relax your chest, neck, shoulders, and face and allow a natural rhythm to develop. Continue for at least 5 minutes, then relax.*

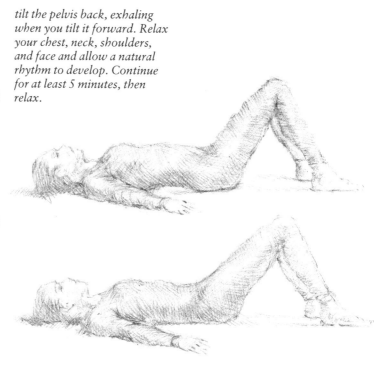

Now imagine a clock face under your pelvis. You have already moved between 12 and 6. Now move between 3 and 9 o'clock, then rotate slowly around the full hour in both a clockwise and anti-clockwise direction. You may find you are prevented by stiffness or tension from making a smooth and full movement in a certain place. If this is the case, spend some time moving just in the quarter or semicircle that includes the tight spot, to loosen it. Keep your breathing regular and rhythmic throughout the movement and don't tighten your buttocks.

Pelvic vibration

Stand in front of a table or heavy chair, feet hip-width apart, and put a cushion (or folded blanket) in front of you. Steadying yourself with your hands, bend your knees and put your weight on the balls of your feet, allowing your heels to come off the floor. Now arch backward, tilting the pelvis back also, and maintain this stance, breathing fully. When your legs start to vibrate, gently thrust your hips back and forth. As the vibrations rise into your pelvis, it may swing back and forth on its own. If your legs feel strained, you can use the cushion to fall on to your knees.

Standing hip rotation
This is the movement that belly
dancers make; practised
regularly it will loosen up the
pelvic area and free the energy
flow in your body.

Stand with your legs apart,
knees slightly bent. Feel your
contact with the ground. Now
put your hands on your hips
and begin to move them
forward and back several
times, then from side to side,
and finally in a wide circle –
forward, right, back, left. Let
your hips, not your legs, direct
the movement and keep your
breathing steady, relaxing your
belly and buttocks.

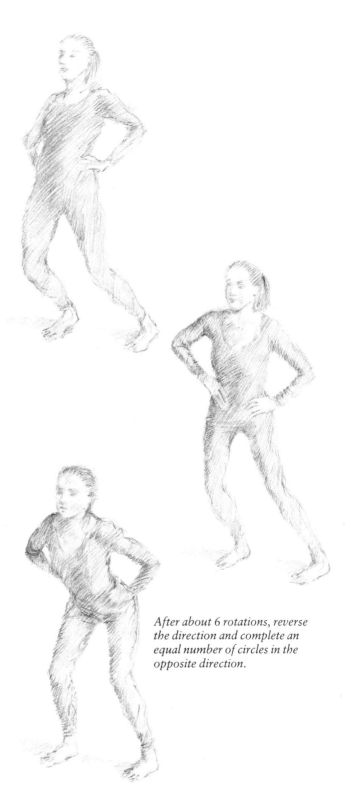

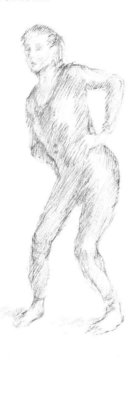

After about 6 rotations, reverse
the direction and complete an
equal number of circles in the
opposite direction.

Sensing

Our senses are our point of contact with the world. They bring us pleasure and pain, experience and information. But much of our sensing ability lies unused below the threshold of our awareness, effectively dormant for long periods of time. We often notice how much sharper the senses of animals seem to be than our own – a cat or dog will respond to sounds we have not heard, investigate smells we cannot distinguish. Many of us, too, have experienced times when our own senses were sharpened. On holiday, in a different climate and a new environment, we hear the sounds of life; we let the colours bathe our eyes, smell the unfamiliar smells and, walking barefoot on the beach, we feel the sand trickle between our toes. At such times we feel relaxed, alive, fully in the "here and now".

In day-to-day life, by contrast, our senses often seem dull, unused, and our experience and contact with present reality seem blunted too. In fact, the senses themselves never cease to pick up and relay floods of information. But we perceive only what we pay attention to, so if our minds are constantly preoccupied, we miss most of the messages of our senses. Our senses are also much affected by our feelings. We may escape, or blunt the edges of, reality by unconsciously dulling the sensitivity of our sense organs – avoiding eye contact, for example, or withdrawing attention from our ears. In addition, our sensory system is tuned to recognize and screen out the normal, familiar stimuli, and to bring to our notice only the unusual, the significant, or maybe the survival-threatening – the foot on the stair, our name spoken in a crowded room, a rotten smell, an unfamiliar taste. This sensory screening is necessary – without it, we would be drowned in the flood of sensation, and find it difficult to cope with daily tasks or, if we live in a city, with the noise and confusion of life. But as a result, the mere pleasure of "being" – walking, eating, touching, really seeing what is around us – often passes us by.

At their full capacity, our senses are extraordinary, finely tuned even to the subtlest of distinctions. We can distinguish between a half- and a quarter-tone in music and, by just touching someone's forehead, tell whether their body temperature is deviating by no more than a degree or two from normal.

This chapter shows you how to develop your sensory awareness through specially selected exercises for each of the senses – sight, touch, smell, hearing, and taste. By increasing your responsiveness and sensitivity, you can open up a whole new sensual way of being, and feel more in touch with the world around you. With a little practice, you can extend what you learn into your everyday activities and, through sharpening your perceptions, and discovering how to experience the present moment, improve your whole quality of life.

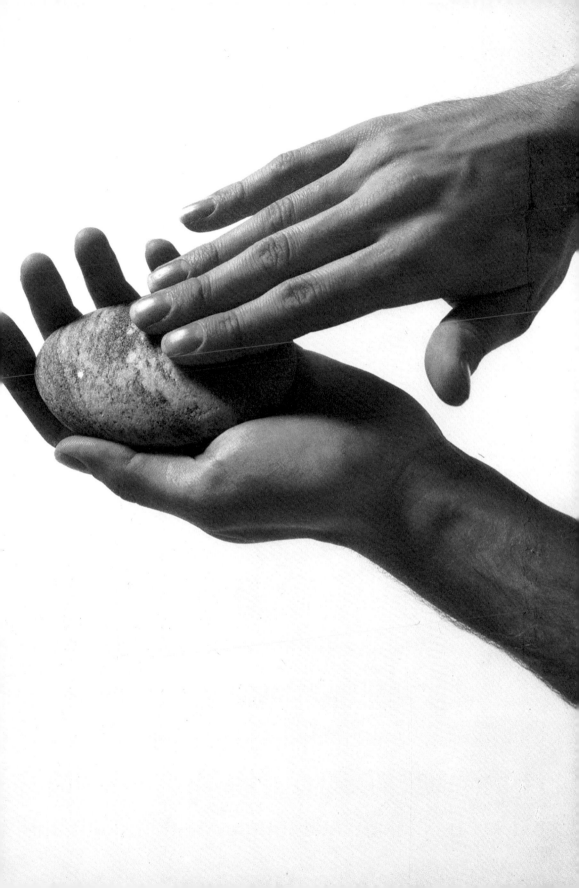

Here and now

Within the wonderful galaxy of sounds, feelings, sights, smells, and perceptions that make up consciousness, our attention shifts constantly – from our immediate "outer" world to the "inner" world of our imagination, with all its plans, thoughts, and memories, that keep us away from the "here and now" of the present. Being fully in the here and now means paying attention to what our senses are telling us, without suppressing the inevitable intrusion of thought, memory, and imagination. Simply choosing to let go of these "inner" thoughts, rather than holding on and getting involved in them, allows you to enjoy ordinary, everyday sensations much more. Being fully in the present moment in this way means being clear about both your "worlds", and knowing which one to respond to. The exercises that follow encourage you to immerse yourself totally in the world of your senses and in the here and now, while doing something as commonplace as washing the dishes. If thoughts and feelings come up, don't waste time criticizing yourself for failing to be in the present; simply let them pass and gently return your attention to what you are doing.

"Attention to sensing quiets what is compulsive in our thought, so that the mind becomes free and available for its normal function of perception. When the radio in the mind is stilled, everything else can come to life."
Charles V. W. Brooks
Sensory Awareness

Washing the dishes
While washing the dishes, see how far you can keep your attention on the sounds you are making, the sloshing of the water, the wet surfaces that you are washing, the feel of the soap suds on your fingers, the smell of the room. Rest your attention lightly on all of this and notice what happens.

Pausing
Pausing or slowing down an everyday activity can provide an excellent opportunity to practise being in the present. We often don't notice the messages from our senses until we slow down or even stop.

While you are involved in an activity, ask someone, or set a timer, to interrupt you after a few minutes. Now check. Where was your attention? On the sensory point of contact? Or on a thought or feeling? If the latter, let go of it without criticism and return to the task, having arranged to be interrupted again.

Painting a wall

Painting a door or a wall is an excellent way of enhancing your ability to get in touch with your senses and practising being in the present moment.

Try to give light but continuous attention to every aspect of the task. Light attention works better than concentration, which implies effort. Feel the weight of the paint in the tin, the pressure on the screwdriver you use to open it. Listen to the sound of the lid coming open, and smell the paint – first in the tin and then on your brush. Keep your attention on the point of contact between the brush and the surface you are painting.

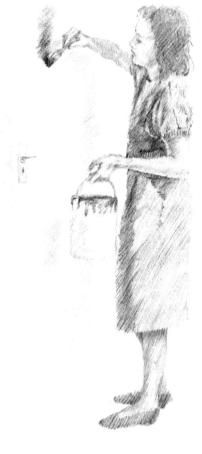

Calligraphy

Bringing the senses into play through working at being in the "here and now" leads to a very calm, relaxed frame of mind. One of the best ways to achieve this calm settling of the senses into the present moment is the practice of calligraphy.

Calligraphers recognize that the quality of drawn letters and words depends on the "here and now" quality of attention in the person doing the work. They also know that the best calligraphy comes from light, steady attention that is unruffled by anxiety or judgements about whether the letters and words are "good" or "bad".

The more you experience the sensory awakening that being in the "here and now" brings, the easier it will become to apply this quality of attention to other areas of life.

Focusing

Practising "focused sensing" enables you to connect quickly with the part of a task that needs attention. You decide which sensations you will let in, and which you can afford to neglect, in the interests of concentrating your awareness. Learning to "selectively neglect" in this way can be vital if you need to hear what someone is saying in a noisy, crowded café, for instance.

Deliberately shutting down one sense can help to bring the other senses more sharply into your awareness. Closing your eyes, for example, helps you to enjoy and focus on the subtle sensations of touch during a massage, or to hear the waves breaking on a shore, the crying of the seagulls. Turning the radio down and asking people to stop talking can help you to "see" better while driving in heavy traffic.

Sight

The eyes are an extension of the brain and, perhaps because we tend to live so much "in our heads", sight is often the dominant sense – even though touch may exceed it for sheer volume of signals to the brain. If you try giving attention only to what your eyes are doing for a minute or two, you will quickly become aware of the way that they ceaselessly jump about from one centre of interest to another, never staying still. What we observe through our eyes is really like a series of "snapshots", but from this collection of impressions we build up an overall picture of what we actually "see" – a whole world of colour, shape, hue, texture, and space. In the exercises that follow, you practise "focused attention", using your eyes to focus on just the edge or outline of an object, and then focusing on the space around it. Take it slowly and don't strain – if you feel your eyes tiring, simply look away, rest, and try again.

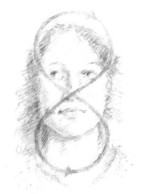

Figure of 8
Imagine a large figure "8" suspended in the air in front of you. Slowly begin to trace its shape with your gaze, until you have outlined a full figure of 8. Trace the 8 several times in each direction.

Edging

Sit comfortably and let your gaze settle on the outline of something fairly simple and strong in shape, like a vase of flowers or a chair.

Now, very slowly, trace the edge of the object with your eyes – don't jump or cheat. Maintain a light steady gaze and don't strain.

Drawing

Focused attention can be directed toward a surface or a space as well as toward an edge. Find a light-coloured object, such as a vase of flowers or an ornament, and place it against a dark background.

Now, with pencil or crayons and paper, try drawing the space around what you have chosen. Try drawing in the large solid areas first and then gradually work your way across to the edges of the object.

Hearing

Our sense of hearing provides us with the greatest capacity for taking in what is happening around us. Without it, we live cut off from the atmosphere that sound can convey – the stillness of a forest clearing, the cacophony of sounds in a city centre, the tremendous gushing of a waterfall. Our hearing, too, has remarkable powers of selective attention, sorting out what we want to hear from what we are content to neglect. Even so, it can be surprisingly difficult to rest our hearing continually on a single sound. The exercise below shows you how to stay with a single source of sound, while keeping it relatively uncontaminated by input from the other senses, or from the mind. The essence of this kind of hearing is to avoid strain, so don't try to empty your mind of everything but what you hear. If thoughts come in, just let go of them, gently returning your attention to the sound.

Glass harmonica
Select 2 good-quality wine glasses. Wash them and your own hands very thoroughly with a mild detergent or shampoo. When they are clean, you should find that stroking around the top edge of the glasses with a wet finger generates a very pure tone as the glass resonates like a violin string.

Now try tuning the glasses to different notes by partly filling them with water, and stroking them again. Keep your attention focused on the pure tones you are making.

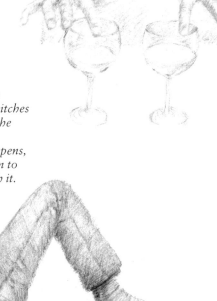

Hearing a line of melody
Choose a piece of solo music to listen to on a record or tape. Jazz solos or classical flute, violin, or piano solos work well. Lie down and close your eyes. If you have earphones, use them.

Now let your hearing rest steadily and persistently on the melodic line, or the sound pattern if it has no melody.

See how long you can go before your attention switches out of the music to 1 of the other senses, or to stray thoughts. When this happens, just return your attention to the melody and stay with it.

Touch

Operating through our skin, our sense of touch provides a vital source of information about our close surroundings, our "state of being", and our contact with reality. It is also a major source of pleasure. People who lack sight or hearing largely rely on exploring and experiencing the world through their sense of touch, and often develop acute sensitivity in their hands. You can explore this yourself, cutting off your sight by blindfolding yourself or just closing your eyes, and simply touching and feeling different textures and shapes, immersing yourself totally in the nuances of sensation. Even everyday tasks, like washing your hair, can be enriched by attending to the "feel" of the whole experience, rather than just doing it mechanically. You can enhance many of the unconsidered humdrum activities of living by focusing on your sense of touch in this way.

Shampooing your hair
When next you wash your hair, try doing it slowly and deliberately. If you usually race through it, take your time and slow down. Enjoy the feel of the foam on your hands, and the sensual rubbing of your hands on your scalp. Pause frequently to give yourself time to register the sensations in your scalp, in your fingertips, in your face, around your eyes.

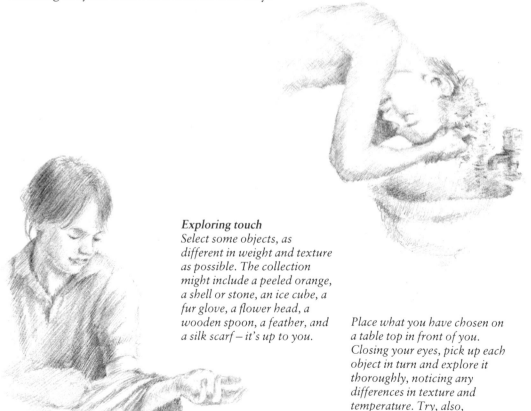

Exploring touch
Select some objects, as different in weight and texture as possible. The collection might include a peeled orange, a shell or stone, an ice cube, a fur glove, a flower head, a wooden spoon, a feather, and a silk scarf – it's up to you.

Place what you have chosen on a table top in front of you. Closing your eyes, pick up each object in turn and explore it thoroughly, noticing any differences in texture and temperature. Try, also, touching different objects and textures with your bare feet.

Taste and smell

Our senses of taste and smell are inextricably linked. Smell something savoury and your mouth begins to water; smell something rotten and you get a bad taste in your mouth. As any cat or dog knows, there is a wealth of things to be smelt and tasted in everyday life – a world of sensation that few of us humans have discovered. It is amazingly therapeutic to come across good smells – forest ferns, freshly baked bread, roasting coffee beans. Smell is the most evocative of senses, changing our mood, and recalling unexpected memories. Yet it is also the most ignored, its powerful messages often passing us by unnoticed.

The same applies to our sense of taste. Most of us only eat to "fill our bellies", not to really experience the richness and variety of taste sensations our food can provide. If we tasted and smelt what we ate consciously, we wouldn't eat as much. Awakening to the power of taste and smell can greatly enhance your life. You can begin to do this by reducing input from the other senses, especially the eyes, and focusing attention on the sense of taste or smell only.

Tasting with awareness
Prepare a meal for yourself in which most of the ingredients remain separate. Then begin to eat the food slowly, savouring the flavour of every mouthful and enjoying the process of biting, chewing, and swallowing. Feel how your teeth and your tongue deal with the food. Pause occasionally as you eat and notice if the taste changes at all as the food is broken down, then slowly swallow. You may be surprised at how full you feel before you get to the end of your plate, when you eat consciously in this way.

Consciously smelling
Gather together some strong-smelling objects – flowers, fresh or dried, herbs, peeled and cut fruit, soap, and so forth. Close your eyes and, picking up 1 object at a time, slowly absorb the fragrance of each one. Try also making a meal on the basis of smell. Include a succession of dishes ranging from pungent to rich, and inhale the smell of each dish before eating it.

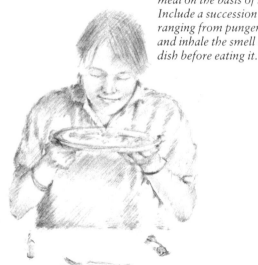

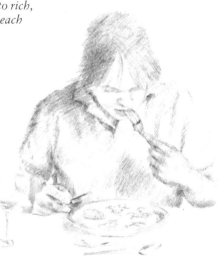

Opening

We often "narrow" our senses to focus on something specific, like reading a book, for example. Although there may be many distractions around us – noises, movements, smells, changes of temperature – we unconsciously screen them out in favour of the task in hand. "Opening" to the whole range of sensory nuances is immensely rewarding, for it gives new zest to activities, situations, or events which might otherwise be considered mundane.

Putting this "opening" into effect involves temporarily letting go of the need to understand or label what is happening and moving toward simply experiencing it, immersing yourself in all the sensory dimensions. By maintaining a "beginner's mind" (see p.34), you give yourself permission to be surprised, to discover anew the value and richness of the "ordinary". Opening yourself up to the full sensory impact of an experience means reducing (but not eliminating) the control of your cognitive mind. Afterward, it's a good idea to spend a little time evaluating how you felt about the experience, and discovering what you learnt from it. In our society, intellect rules with an iron hand. Experiencing in an open rather than a focused way has the special value of uniting thinking and feeling.

Open seeing

We all possess a very wide field of vision, but can only focus precisely on one small area at a time. Learning to become aware of and give your attention to your outer or peripheral vision, gives you a new and interesting perspective on reality. It leads to you valuing what you may only be dimly aware of "out of the corner of your eye", and learning to have "eyes in the back of your head", so that you can pick up the inconsequential details of people's behaviour which, taken as a whole, may be sending messages too subtle for verbal definition.

Drawing the whole field of vision
With a large sheet of paper and some coloured pens or crayons, use your left hand (if right-handed) to make a drawing of the totality of what you can see when you give attention to your peripheral vision. Do whatever it takes to suggest the whole field of your vision, concentrating on giving an impression of your extended view rather than on any specific details.

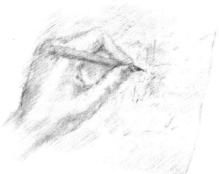

Open hearing

Opening your hearing to experience the whole range and variety of sound vibrations around you means moving away from listening for melody, harmony, speech, or song, toward an appreciation of the abundance of different noises.

Because they all invite recognition in some way, melody, harmony, and speech pull the mind toward understanding or judging what you are hearing. Temporarily suspending these judgements will have the effect of opening up your listening to include the noise of the wind in the trees, of crows fighting over a tasty morsel, of the swish of a car passing by, rain on an umbrella, or your shoes crunching through snow. You may find yourself less likely to regard noise as an irritation, or a weed in the garden of sounds.

Street market
Part of the reason why street markets such as this one continue to be so popular is that they appeal to all our senses. Next time you go to a market, enjoy really smelling the cooking food, the ripe vegetables, and notice the continual movement of people, the range of shapes, colours, and textures. Immerse yourself totally in the irresistible mix of sensory pleasures.

Hearing into the distance
Sit comfortably, near a window. Close your eyes, and remain very still and quiet, until you can hear the noise in your own head (a very faint shushing sound). Open your listening to include sounds in the room, too. Follow this by including the sounds in the street outside. Finally, open your listening to include the most distant sounds.

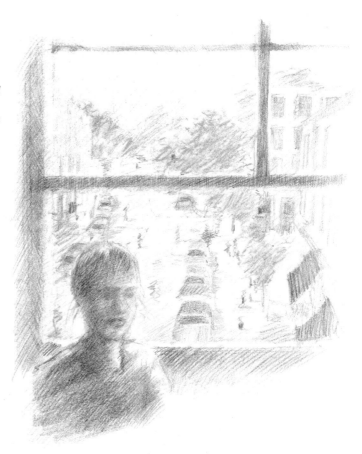

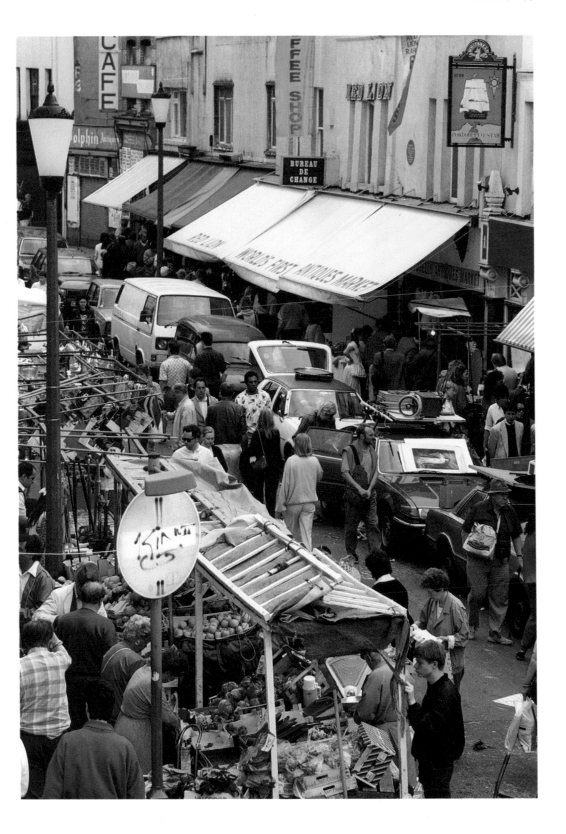

Self-assessment

Being fully aware means having access to all our ways of sensing. But being human, we need to accept that some of our senses will be more developed, more open, than others.

When you have had some practice in experiencing through your senses, you may find it useful to assess where your strengths and weaknesses are in this area, so that you can take action to remedy any imbalance that you discover.

A useful approach to assessing yourself is to set a modest goal of, each day, shifting a small piece of your life into experiencing mode. For instance, try plunging totally into the action of walking home from work, or shopping, or walking the dog. Avoid making any judgements during this period. Then when you have the opportunity, shift out of the experiencing mode and consider what happened. How did you feel about it? Was one of your senses dominating? Would you do it any differently next time?

Assessment exercise
Each day, write down under a series of headings, 1 for each of the senses, what sensations you experienced that day.

If, after a while, you find that 1 or 2 columns are beginning to be full, while others are almost empty of entries, you will know which of your senses are in play and which are not.

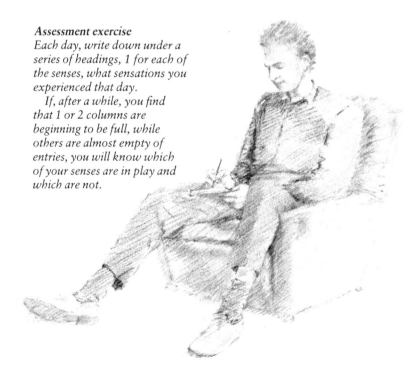

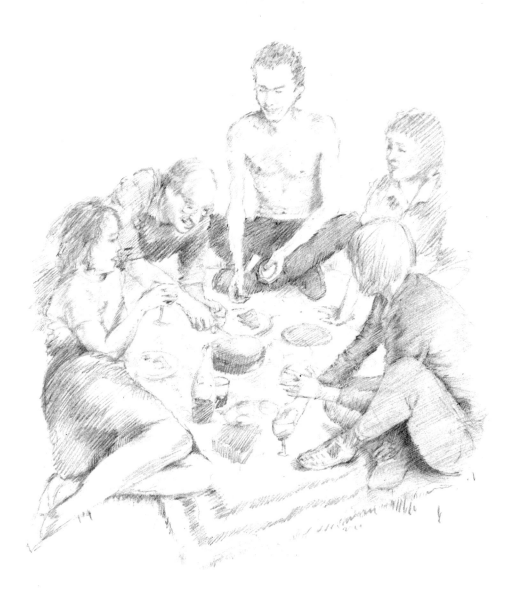

Picnic

Once the value and interest of extended sensing has been realized, you can take the opportunity to exercise it when suitable events arise. Picnics are a good example, for the ingredients of a good picnic are those which excite the senses.

We usually sit on the ground, and eat with our fingers. We are likely to wear less clothes than usual, and be exposed to the wind and the sunshine. Often we run, play games, and generally "fool about".

Yet were you to ask each of the people at the picnic what made the greatest impression on them, you would probably have as many answers as there are people, such is the diversity and richness of the human sensory mix.

Celebrating the earth
African dance

Learning to dance is an exciting way of discovering how to use our bodies to express our feelings by creating patterns of movement. We have all danced at some time, but for many of us it is an all too rare occurrence. In Africa, however, dance is an integral part of daily life: from formal dances at important ceremonies to informal celebrations where everyone dances together.

African styles of dance differ from those familiar to us. The dancers follow the dictates of their musical rhythms allowing the music to flow through their bodies with a sensual ease. They accept their bodies positively, dancing with confidence and expressive skill to the percussive beat. In our society we lack this ease, but learning African dance will enable you to move with style to the subtle rhythms of Africa.

In this chapter we present some dance postures and movements for you to learn, so you can begin to experience a new freedom of expression as you move to the rhythmic beat. With practice, your movements will become more earth-centered as you gain the balance between control and relaxation that frees you to enjoy dancing to African music.

African dance offers you a way of discovering the movement rhythms of your own body. As you allow yourself to feel the pulse of the drums by shifting your weight from one foot to the other, you learn to accept the weight of your body, in a repetitive rhythmic return to the earth. These skills enable you to be at home in your body – to walk and move with an ease which unites your mental and physical energies. By mastering the art, you experience a new freedom and spontaneity of movement. Through the rhythmic patterns and gestures, you can express the "intention" of your dance, which gives a sense of meaning to your movements.

For the people of Africa, dance is a celebration of their way of life, expressing their relationship with the community, and with their protective spirits. The dance patterns grow out of the rhythms of their natural environment, their manual work, and their everyday movement habits. Music and dance are central to ritual ceremonies, marriages, funerals, and all important social events in the community. Although skilled dancers perform at ceremonies, there is always a time for everyone to dance for pleasure. No one is too fat, too old, or too crippled to join the dance in their own way, for the dancers accept their own being, experiencing themselves as a unity of mind, body, and spirit.

Performing African dance away from this environment naturally results in changes of style, but as you dance to celebrate a return to the earth you will discover that it enables you to express yourself as a whole person – a valuable gift which is all too rare in our fragmented, fast-moving society.

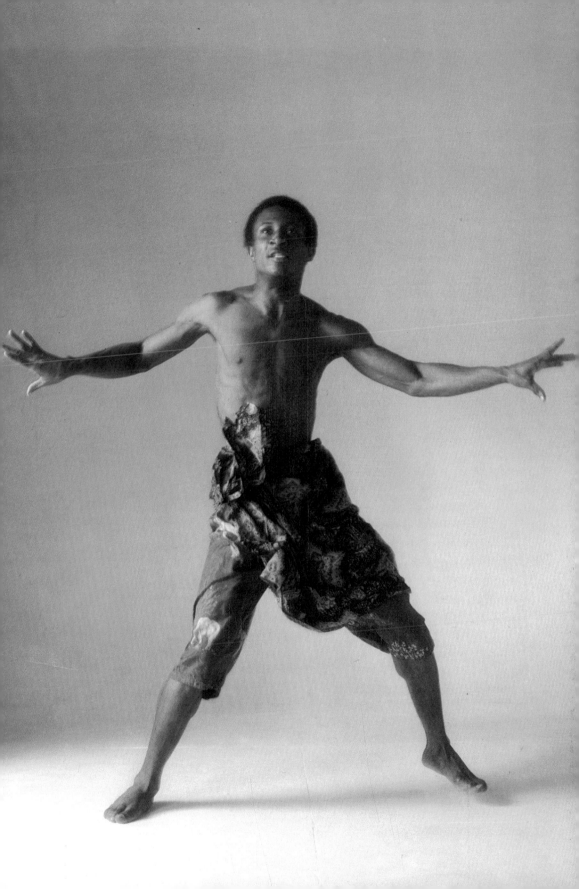

The elements of African dance

Before attempting the exercises and dance movements that follow, you need to understand the basic principles of African dance and the ideas that motivate the dancers, for their dance is an expression of their way of life.

Dance entails moving through space and using time to express an idea or an emotion. Western dance is primarily concerned with space, but in African dance the time element of rhythm is the dominant factor. The skill of African dancers is judged on their ability to move to the rhythm of the drums with precision and subtlety.

Posture is all-important in African dance, and there are three main postures to learn – the upright, the inclined, and the deeply inclined posture (see pp.90-3). Your weight is centered in your hips and directed down into the earth through the rhythmic movements of your knees and feet. This gives you a firm basis for holding a strong, straight back, and flattening the small of your back, to allow for the characteristic backward thrust of the buttocks. You use your knees as springs for the rhythmic transference of your weight from one part of the body to the other, which creates a balance of weight in your body.

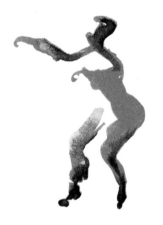

Your hips are the centre of control for your upper body, which should remain poised but relaxed. As in all dance, it is essential to have a sense of your body centre, from which all your movements and your breathing are controlled.

Isolation of movement is an important element of African dance. It means being able to isolate shoulder or hip patterns while keeping your torso still. The part of the body that is isolated varies: the Ijo women use a deeply inclined posture which frees their hips to vibrate to the drum rhythms; the Ika use strong pelvic contractions in their erotic courtship dances; the Yoruba people use both hip and shoulder patterns, but never at the same time, as this would hamper the flow of rhythm.

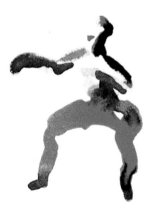

Gestures in dance can be performed with any part of the body not supporting your weight. You speak through your gestures, as when you embrace and draw strength from the earth in the Tiv women's dance, and when you energetically flourish your horsetail switch to express your delight in the Irigwe farmers' dance.

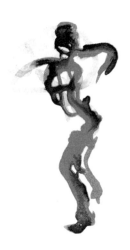

"Progression" describes the way you move from one place to another; it varies greatly in different dance styles. The Irigwe farmers, for instance, dance in a circle, using rapid hops and jumps to encourage their crops to grow. The Ijo people dance in lines, allowing soloists to emerge with rapid staccato foot rhythms – movements which reflect balancing in their canoes or wading through their flooded villages. The Tiv women's confident stance comes from farming the solid earth of the open savannah. Yoruba dancers move freely amongst each other, as though weaving through the dense forests which surround their villages.

Throughout Africa the temperament of the people is expressed in their dance. Ijo men are fierce fighters and dance to rapidly accelerating tempos in short intense dances, whereas the Kambari repeat a simple rhythm at a steady tempo throughout the night.

In the vast continent of Africa there are thousands of different styles of dance, but they are all based on percussive rhythmic patterns which repeatedly return to the earth.

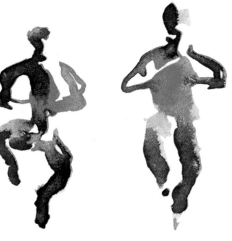

Preparing to dance

To do the following rhythmic exercises, we recommend that you obtain some form of percussive music to guide your movements and allow you to "feel" the rhythm with your body. In Africa, the rhythmic music creates an atmosphere which invites you to dance. You may know someone who plays a drum or a tambourine. Otherwise, find a store which sells African music. Ask for a four-beat rhythm, a two-four-beat rhythm, and a three-beat rhythm. A four-beat rhythm puts the accent on the first of four beats, a two-four beat accents the first and third of four beats, and a three-beat rhythm accents the third of three beats. Before beginning to move, internalize the rhythm by singing it to yourself. Wear loose, comfortable clothing that does not restrict your movements in any way. Working in bare feet is best, for it allows you to feel the surface on which you are dancing with your whole foot. Dance on an even surface in or out of doors, and avoid slippery surfaces. You may practise alone, but since African dance is communal, it would be more fun to dance with friends, as you could help each other to hold the postures and perform the rhythm with precision.

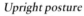

Upright posture
Stand with your feet shoulder-width apart, knees relaxed. Concentrate your control in your hips, keeping the small of your back straight, your spine stretching upright into your neck. Your head remains easily poised, your upper body and arms relaxed. Now, bending your elbows slightly, bring your hands up to the sides of your hips with palms facing down. Feel your body weight becoming centered down into the earth.

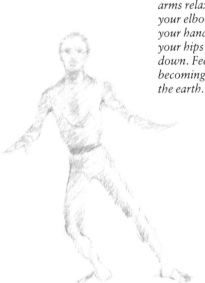

Shoulder beats
Play a repetitive 4-beat rhythm with a steady tempo. Taking the upright posture, begin to raise and drop your shoulders to the beat of the rhythm, developing a steady percussive beat. Now, keeping your heels on the floor, transfer your weight to your right foot, drawing your upright body sideways, with your shoulders parallel to the floor, still keeping the shoulder beat going. Repeat this movement to the left. Use 4 shoulder beats in each direction.

Shoulder rolls

Keeping your feet firmly on the
ground, perform a continuous
circular movement by lifting
your shoulders one at a time,
then rolling them back down
and to the front to 4 beats.
Later, try 2 rolls to 4 beats.

Rhythmic transfer of weight through the knees

Play a 2/4-beat rhythm. Take
the upright posture, feeling the
rhythm by transferring your
weight – through your knees –
from 1 foot to the other with
the beat. As you shift your
weight on to the right foot,
your right knee becomes
straight but not locked, and
the left knee remains relaxed.
The reverse happens when you
shift to the left. Keep your
heels on the floor and your
head at a steady level. Then
accent the rhythm with a
double beat of the supporting
knee on each side.

Rhythmic transfer of weight through the hips

With the same rhythm playing,
starting from the upright
posture, shift your weight from
left to right through your hips.
Push your hips to the right,
your right leg straightening as
it takes the weight – the left
knee remains relaxed. Repeat
to the left. Bend your elbows,
making sure your hands are
relaxed. Now, keeping your
heels on the ground, swing
your weight in your hips from
side to side with a double beat
on each side.

Inclined posture with hip beats
*Bend your knees and push out
your buttocks behind you,
bending your back forward
about 30 degrees from the
upright. Keep your neck on a
line with your spine and your
gaze directed toward the floor.
Bending your elbows back
behind your torso, leave your
hands in front, with palms
upward on either side of your
waist. Shift your weight to
your right hip by straightening
your right knee, keeping your
left knee bent. Repeat this to
the left.*

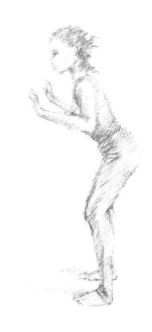

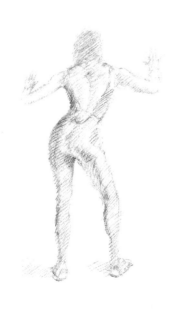

*Now, to a 2/4-beat rhythm,
begin swinging your buttocks
rhythmically from side to side,
with a double beat on each
side, as you isolate your hip
movements from your upper
body. When confident, you can
double the tempo of your hip
swing.*

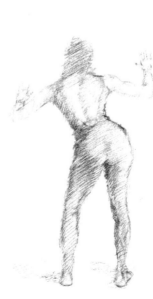

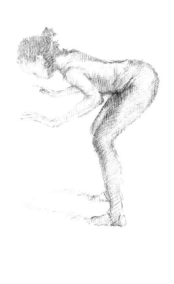

Deeply inclined posture (based on Ijo women's dance)

Stand with your feet 18 inches apart, knees relaxed. Place your hand on the small of your back to ensure that it is flat and, moving from this point, bring your upper back down until your torso is parallel to the floor. Hold your back straight, extending into the line of your neck, so that you are looking straight down on to the floor. Thrust your buttocks out at the back, bringing your weight on to the balls of your feet without raising your heels.

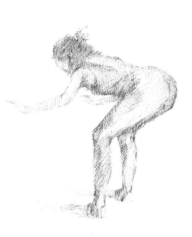

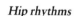

Hip rhythms

Playing a 2/4-beat rhythm, turn your knees toward the body centre as this produces a roll in the hips to right and left. Accent the double beat to each side. As you master this movement the rhythmic pattern becomes concentrated in the roll of the hips and buttocks until you are able to perform with a minimum of leg movement.

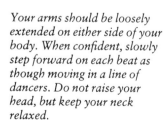

Your arms should be loosely extended on either side of your body. When confident, slowly step forward on each beat as though moving in a line of dancers. Do not raise your head, but keep your neck relaxed.

Circle dance (based on Irigwe farmers' dance)

The circle is a familiar image in African dance – the people's beliefs are based on reincarnation, which recognizes a continuous cycle of life and death.

Imagine you are one of a team of dancers moving sideways along a circular floor pattern around drummers who play a 3-beat rhythm. Assume the inclined posture and bring your weight on to the balls of your feet, with heels slightly raised. Begin to move anti-clockwise, as follows:

Beat 1 Step right and lift the left foot, bending your left knee.

Beat 2 Hop on the right foot, holding your left foot.

Beat 3 Place your left foot next to the right foot and perform a neat jump on the spot, with feet together and knees forward.

Repeat this 3-beat pattern 3 times and add a second pattern of 3 neat jumps, with your feet together and your knees up. When you have mastered this pattern, add 3 shoulder beats to coincide with the beats of the 3 jumps. The complete dance pattern is performed to 4 repeats of the 3-beat musical pattern. The Irigwe farmers carry a horsetail whisk in their right hands, which they may flourish to the rhythm.

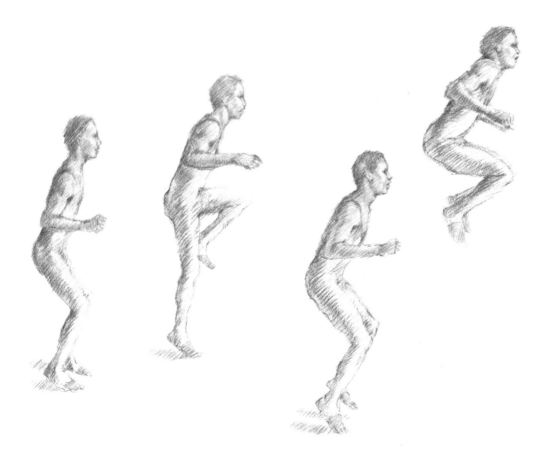

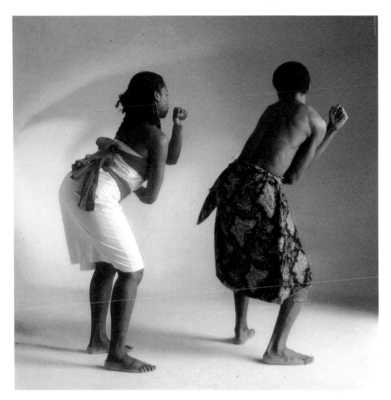

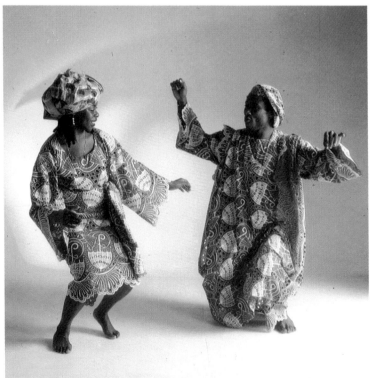

Circle dance (based on Tiv women's dance)
This dance is performed from a static position using a slow sustained movement. Stand with your heels about 18 inches apart, your feet slightly turned out.

A. Perform the dance pattern to a 2 x 4-beat rhythm – this has 8 beats.

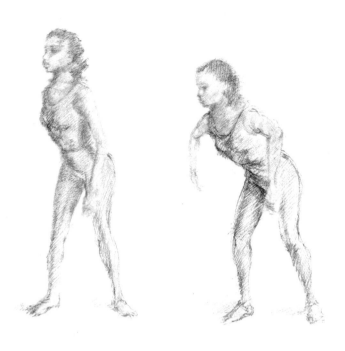

Beats 1,2 Bend both knees deeply, with feet staying flat on the floor, torso slightly inclined. As your knees bend, slowly raise your elbows in line with your shoulders...

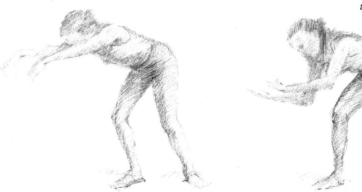

...Transferring your weight to your right foot and knee, turn your torso to incline slightly to the right. As it turns, extend your arms into a loose curve, using soft hands with palms down beyond your bowed head.

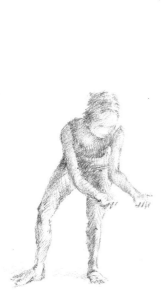
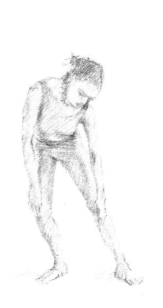
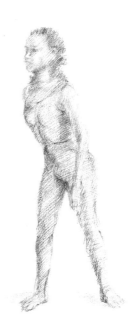

Beats 3,4 Transfer your weight on to your left knee and hip, drawing your inclined torso over to the left. Turn your palms loosely upward and draw your hands across the body to the left, following your torso.

Beats 5,8 Recover the upright position as the rhythm flows through your body, and sway from the left foot to the right and back to the left in preparation for the next move.

After performing this pattern twice to the right and twice to the left, continue as follows:

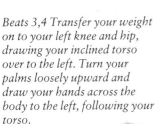
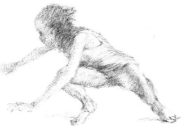

B. Beats 1,2 Bend both knees into a deep squat, with your torso slightly inclined, feet flat or with heels slightly raised and head bowed. Move your arms loosely to the right.

Beats 3,4 Brush your hands lightly above the surface of the floor.

Beats 5,6 Move your arms loosely to the left side, to allow your hands to perform the brushing gesture to the left.

Beat 7 Move your arms and hands to the right.

Beat 8 Regain standing position, allowing the rhythm to flow smoothly throughout your body. Your head follows the movement of your upper body.

This dance pattern requires the 8-beat rhythm to repeat 3 times. Perform pattern repeatedly for 5 minutes.

Remember to relax and shake out your legs and arms after each exercise.

Inhabiting the body
T'ai chi

Before we can truly feel with our bodies, we first have to learn to inhabit them. In the East there are many disciplines designed to achieve this, but one – T'ai chi – stands out in particular. T'ai chi is an ancient Chinese exercise system rooted in Taoist philosophy, whose origins stretch back at least 4,000 years. Though it belongs to the martial arts, it is more often practised as a form of meditation in movement. *Chi* is the life force or vital energy that permeates the universe and circulates continuously in channels or meridians throughout the body. Practising T'ai chi reconnects you to the flow of universal energy in nature, bringing you back in touch with the flow of universal energy in yourself. By a master, it is ultimately practised as a prayer or a celebration of life.

Beautiful to do as well as to observe, T'ai chi is essentially a flowing succession of movements, striking in their apparent simplicity and effortlessness. The movements co-ordinate body, breath, and awareness and are characterized by a continual shifting of weight and a powerfully expressive use of gesture. Exactness of posture, movement, and gesture are emphasized, not for their own sake, but because precision of movement signifies that you are doing T'ai chi in the right spirit, and with the proper awareness.

By contrast with most western sports and fitness techniques, which work on building muscular power and reshaping the body from the outside, T'ai chi is an "internal" system of exercise in the sense that it concentrates on the need to integrate body and mind, to reshape the body from within, through our inner awareness.

The slowness of movement that is T'ai chi's hallmark encourages receptivity to how the body feels, allowing you to get in touch with yourself. Through observing the way you stand, move, and breathe, you can unlearn unnatural habits and awkwardness, and rediscover a more balanced and integrated way of being. For T'ai chi is not something you "master". It's a constant process of learning about yourself, and unless you retain this "beginner's mind" (see p.34), it will not grant you the quality of experience that is its essence. The real masters of T'ai chi regard themselves as perpetual beginners.

Classically, T'ai chi consists of two "forms" or sequences of movements – one that is more protracted, the "long form", with over one hundred and twenty movements, the other, the "short form", with under forty. But to learn these, you need careful and extended tuition from a T'ai chi master, in the form of regular classes. In this chapter, therefore, we have selected a series of simple exercises designed to introduce you to the path of T'ai chi – to the feeling of inhabiting your body and to the awareness this brings.

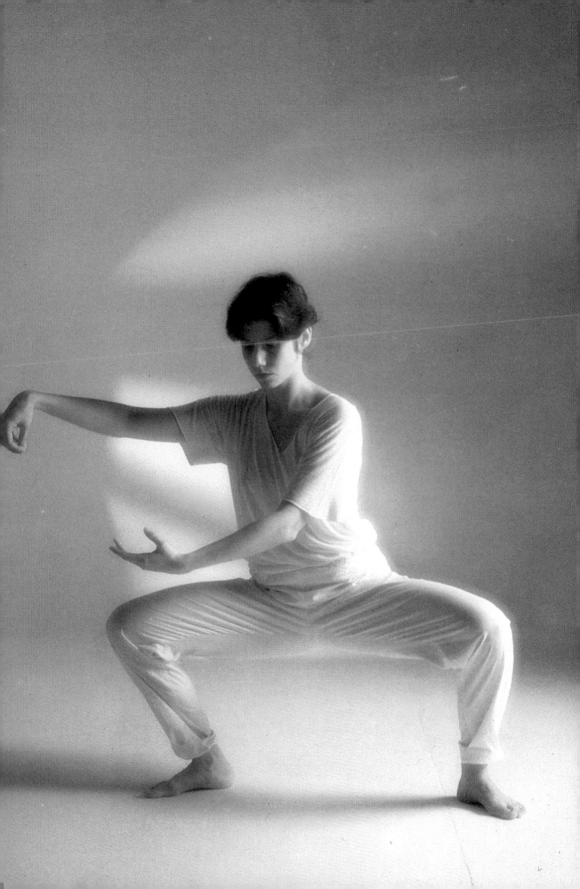

Elements

Before exploring how T'ai chi can help you to come more in touch with yourself, it's important to have an understanding of some of its basic principles.

One of the greatest challenges in T'ai chi is learning to "inhabit" or "own" your body. It is said that if the mind cannot clearly conceive the movement to be performed, then the movement cannot be made. But once there is harmony of intention and movement, then you can even obtain the benefits of the movements simply by imagining yourself doing them.

T'ai chi teaches you to stand and move naturally and breathe from the belly rather than the chest, allowing *chi* to circulate freely. In the T'ai chi classics it is said that: "the intention directs the *chi* and the *chi* directs the body". Although all our everyday movements are preceded by intention, here the use of the mind is made more conscious. In T'ai chi you deliberately use your awareness or intention to direct your energy and guide your body. Ultimately this mental control becomes second nature, resulting in a unique harmony of body and mind, and a rare spontaneity and naturalness of movement.

"It is not wise to rush about, controlling the breath causes strain,
if too much energy is used, exhaustion follows.
This is not the way of Tao."
Tao Te Ching: Lao Tzu

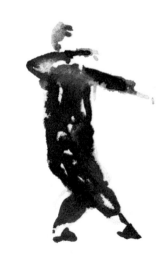

Effortlessness and slowness

For anyone watching T'ai chi in action, one of the most striking features is its apparent effortlessness. When practised by a master, the movements are so slow and fluid that they look like swimming in air. Making the proper movements, however, demands using just the right amount of energy. If you use too much or try too hard, you will force the movement, an approach that is totally alien to the principles of the art. For T'ai chi is a prime example of the Taoist principle of *wu-wei* or non-doing, of going with the flow. To practise it correctly, you need in some way to become childlike, to drop your guard. By making your body as soft and supple as possible, you can move with the minimum of effort.

Of central importance in T'ai chi is the slowness of
the movement. Moving slowly means you need to
inhabit your body continuously, involving yourself
totally in each movement. If you are not fully present,
you won't be able to keep to a slow steady pace, or to
stand still for long. Likewise, if you are feeling
stressed or your mind is over-active, you will find it
hard to move slowly. But if you can persevere and
relax into absorbing yourself in the movement, your
restless mind will eventually quieten, allowing you to
experience a wonderful sense of unity.

Moving with centre

Moving slowly is also the best training for centering
or focusing yourself. Centering means resting your
mind on the *tan t'ien*, the centre of energy in the
abdomen, a few inches below the navel. The *tan t'ien*
(known in Japanese as the *hara*) is the body's centre
of gravity and stability, the centre from which all
movement in the body originates and the meeting
point for body and mind. It is commonly considered
the "earth" centre, for it gathers energy from the
earth rising up through the legs. T'ai chi teaches you
to find and maintain your centre through movement,
whereas in Zen meditation or yoga, centering is
found in stillness. Being centered in the *tan t'ien*
allows you to operate intuitively, with awareness, and
to channel your energy throughout your body.

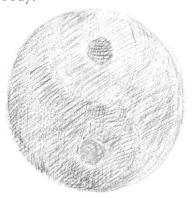

Yin *and* Yang
*Many of the concepts
underlying T'ai chi derive from
an understanding of the need
to balance the complementary
qualities of energy described by
the Chinese as* yin *and* yang *—
qualities of levity and gravity,
for example, or fullness and
emptiness.*

Beginning T'ai chi

When starting T'ai chi, it's best to begin with simple exercises, exploring how your body feels both in stillness and in movement. Here, we have concentrated on teaching just a few basic principles of standing and moving so that you can begin to feel what it's like to inhabit your body with your awareness. At first you may find it easier to experience your body from within if you keep your eyes closed, but your aim should be to maintain an awareness of your body with open eyes. Keep your breathing relaxed, coming from your *tan t'ien* in the lower belly, and don't try too hard. By freeing yourself from self-criticism and accepting yourself as you are, you will begin much sooner to loosen yourself from old patterns of posture and movement and discover your own natural co-ordination and grace. Wear loose clothes to do the exercises and practise them in a well-ventilated room or, better still, out of doors.

Walking forward
Walk very slowly and deliberately around the room, transferring your weight gradually from one foot to the other. Watch how your big toes come off the floor. Become aware of your body travelling through space in one unit, and touch the floor with your feet as if you like it, rather than just using it to pass over.

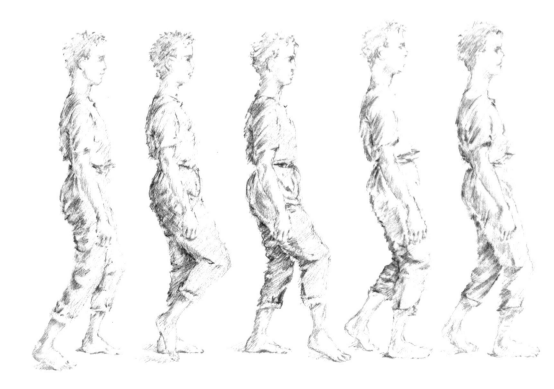

Meditative walking

Slowing down an everyday movement is a valuable
way of establishing whether or not you can truly
inhabit your body. If you feel bored or irritated when
you try this meditative walking, it's a sign that you
are not allowing your awareness to rest in the
movement. If you persevere with walking, however,
you may find that your busy mind gradually desists
from bothering you and you can enjoy the meditative
movement and bask in the feeling of calm it gives you.
Don't mistake this slow deliberate walk for a light
fairylike movement nor for a lazy shuffling step.
Lower your centre of gravity and as you step slowly
forward or backward, feel the foot that bears your
weight becoming heavy and "full", as the other foot
becomes light and "empty".

Walking backward
*Reverse the movement, slowly
placing one foot behind the
other. As one foot fills with
gravity, the other one begins to
come off the floor, ready to
step backward. Keep the
movement smooth.*

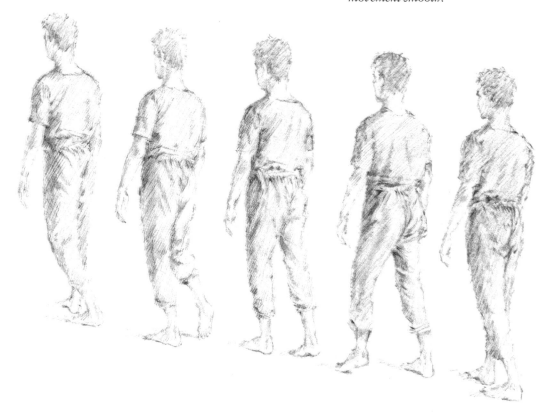

Posture

Your posture is a reflection of your whole way of being. It betrays how you stand in life and how you confront the world – whether you assume a retiring attitude, for instance, holding back from life, or stand tall, facing it squarely. You can't change bad postural habits by trying to be different, however, by copying someone else or emulating a particular body image. You need to experience from inside how different it feels to stand well.

Here we look at basic posture, the starting point for any T'ai chi movements, for before you can move freely and naturally, you need to be able to stand properly, with an awareness of your centre and your position in space. A "good" posture always contains the potential for movement within it, while a "bad" posture is static and stiff. You can discover this for yourself by exploring the extremes of bad posture, as shown below. In either of the two extremes (tense or collapsed), your potential for movement feels constricted, your energy blocked, whereas in the "middle" position, between the extremes, your mobility and energy are freed.

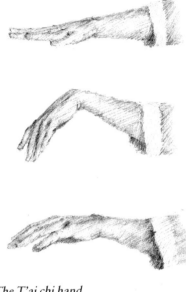

The T'ai chi hand
In T'ai chi, you are constantly endeavouring to find the midpoint between 2 extremes, harmonizing yin and yang. In common with other parts of your body, the hand should be neither tense and stiff nor collapsed and lifeless, but relaxed and open.

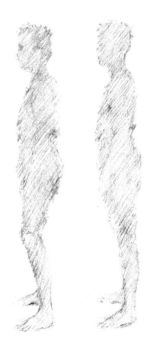

Standing
Stand with your feet pelvis-width apart. Distribute your weight evenly on the triangles made by your heels and the metatarsal joints beneath your big and little toes. Let the soles of your feet feel the floor they are standing on.

Now, to find the best posture for yourself, experiment with the extremes of tension and collapse, focusing in turn on the legs, pelvis, and head. In both extremes you feel stuck, constricted. Try standing with your knees locked, then contrast this by bending them, collapsing down, as shown left. Now find the midway point, where your legs feel ready for movement.

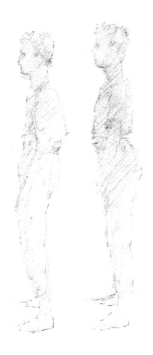

Next, move your attention to the pelvis. Tilt it backward, as far as it will go, then right forward, as shown left. Again, find a place between the 2 extremes. Finally, focus your attention on your head. Pull your chin in toward your throat, then try thrusting it forward. Between these 2 extremes you will find the midpoint where your head sits naturally in line with your spine (right).

Correct posture
Once you have discovered a way of standing that feels effortless and free, explore how your body feels inside.

Try to imagine the floor rising toward you and press down against it with your feet; imagine the ceiling pressing down on you and push up against it with your head. Imagining resistance from above and below gives you a feeling of extension and space between the vertebrae, allowing you to experience your true height. Your upper body (from the tan t'ien up) is like the stem of a flower, growing up toward the light, and your lower body is like the roots, growing down into the earth.

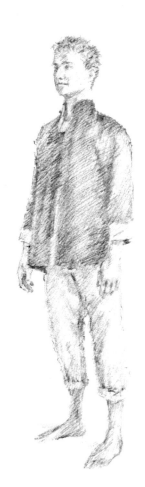

Breathe from the tan t'ien, allowing your mind to rest there. By bringing your attention into your body, you will loosen the control of your brain, break free of the chatter of your busy mind.

Standing like a tree

Trees stand firm in wind and weather, relying on deep roots to keep them earthed. To create the same rootedness and stability in your own body, you need to develop strength in your legs and a strong centre in your *tan t'ien*. For this posture (also called the Riding position), separate your legs wide and bend them, rather than keeping them straight, for by lowering your centre of gravity you come closer to the earth and increase your capacity for stillness and balance. Standing like a tree also makes it easier for you to relax your back and keep it straight. When you stand upright, your back may be hollow or rounded, but in bending your knees, you rely on the strength of your legs to support you and don't need to strain to hold your spine up. Once again, the upper part of your body feels released and light in the position, while the lower half opens to the feeling of heaviness. At first, the position may feel strenuous but once you begin to enjoy the stability it gives you, you'll find you want to stay in it longer and longer as a form of meditation.

Standing like a tree
Stand with your legs more than shoulder-width apart, feet pointing slightly outward. Bend your knees to the point where you can hold the posture without straining. Distribute your weight evenly on both feet, as before. Keeping your spine and head erect, feel the line of gravity passing through you to the centre of the earth. Now bring your arms up as if in an embrace, and join your fingertips in front of your chest, as shown in the photograph, facing page. Rest your attention in the tan t'ien *and watch your breath as it flows softly in and out.*

Turning
Assume the basic position, shown above, but instead of standing still, slowly turn from side to side, letting your waist initiate the movement.

Allow your legs to be "soft", so that they follow the movement led by your waist and let your gaze travel slowly across an imagined horizon.

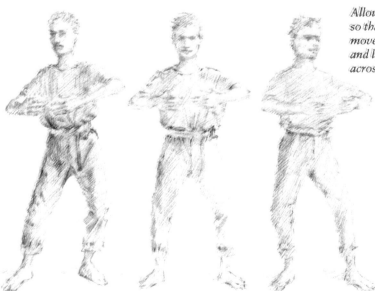

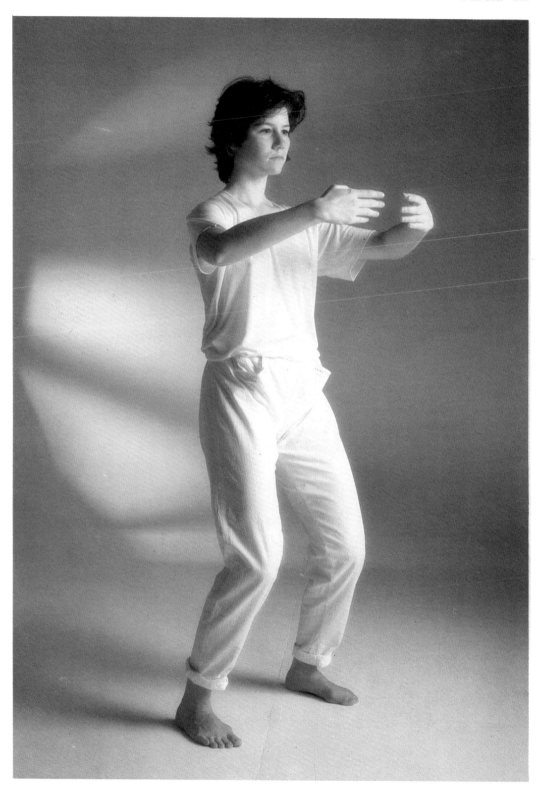

Tree on an abyss

A more powerful way of experiencing rootedness is to
stand on one leg only, allowing yourself to feel the
pull of gravity as if your body were rooted to the
earth through this one leg. This sense of rootedness
allows the rest of the body to resist whatever force
may try to overcome it, even the most powerful wind,
as shown below. If you yield to the feeling of gravity
and keep your attention on the *tan t'ien*, you will not
lose your balance. If you do fall, be aware that it's not
your leg that is weak but the quality of your
attention. Explore this theme of rootedness further by
drawing circles in the air with your weightless leg, as
shown right. Here, once again, your ability to enjoy
freedom of movement lies in the firmness of your
rooted leg which allows the weightless leg to move
effortlessly.

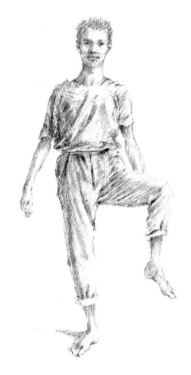

Rooted circles
*Stand on 1 leg and root
yourself firmly to the ground.
Now rotate your free ankle a
few times in 1 direction, then
in the other, drawing circles
with your big toe, as shown
above. Try this also circling
your leg from below the knee
joint, making light, effortless
circles. Then try rotating the
hip joint, bending your leg and
bringing it up toward your
chest and letting your knee
draw circles in the air.*

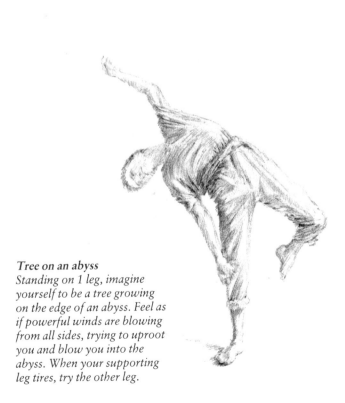

Tree on an abyss
*Standing on 1 leg, imagine
yourself to be a tree growing
on the edge of an abyss. Feel as
if powerful winds are blowing
from all sides, trying to uproot
you and blow you into the
abyss. When your supporting
leg tires, try the other leg.*

Waving hands like clouds

In the world of nature, everything that is alive is in
continuous motion. T'ai chi teaches you to disengage
yourself from the tight control of your judgemental
thinking, allowing you to move freely and
unselfconsciously. In Waving hands like clouds, each
hand in turn symbolically draws energy up from the
tan t'ien, then rotates outward and sinks back down
to where it started. As each palm rises to the level of
your eyes, you rest your gaze on it, turning your head
to follow it until it begins to sink and your attention
moves to the other palm. Inhabit the movement with
awareness, keeping the flow smooth and continuous.

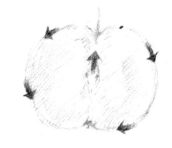

*It may help you to understand
the movement if you think of
an apple cut in half. The core
of the apple is your spine and
the two overlapping circles
trace the movement of your
hands.*

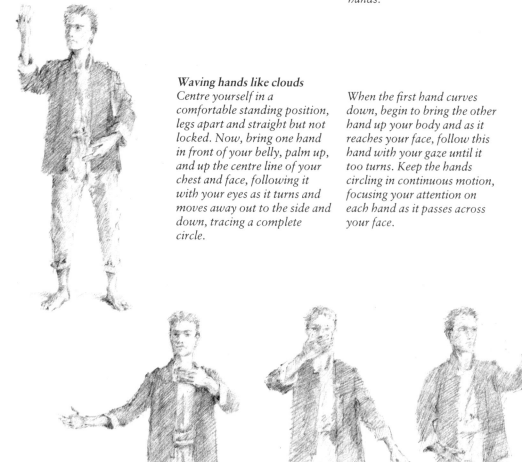

Waving hands like clouds
*Centre yourself in a
comfortable standing position,
legs apart and straight but not
locked. Now, bring one hand
in front of your belly, palm up,
and up the centre line of your
chest and face, following it
with your eyes as it turns and
moves away out to the side and
down, tracing a complete
circle.*

*When the first hand curves
down, begin to bring the other
hand up your body and as it
reaches your face, follow this
hand with your gaze until it
too turns. Keep the hands
circling in continuous motion,
focusing your attention on
each hand as it passes across
your face.*

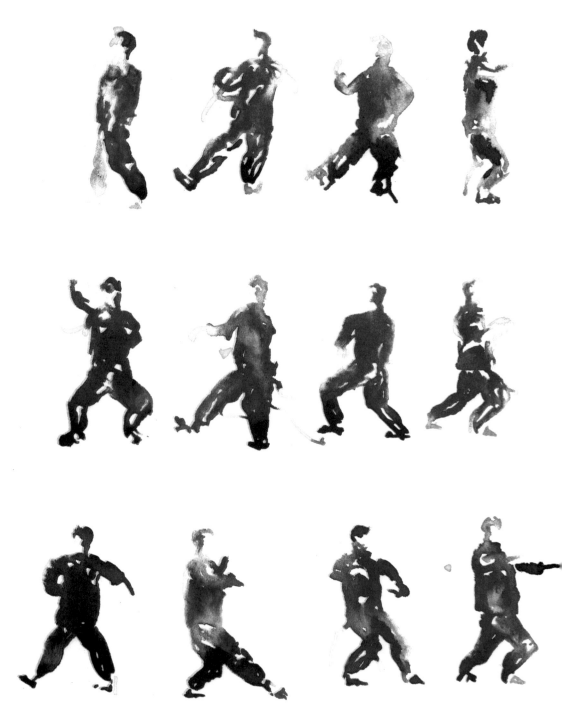

"Be as still as a mountain
move like a great river".
Lao Tzu: Tao Te Ching

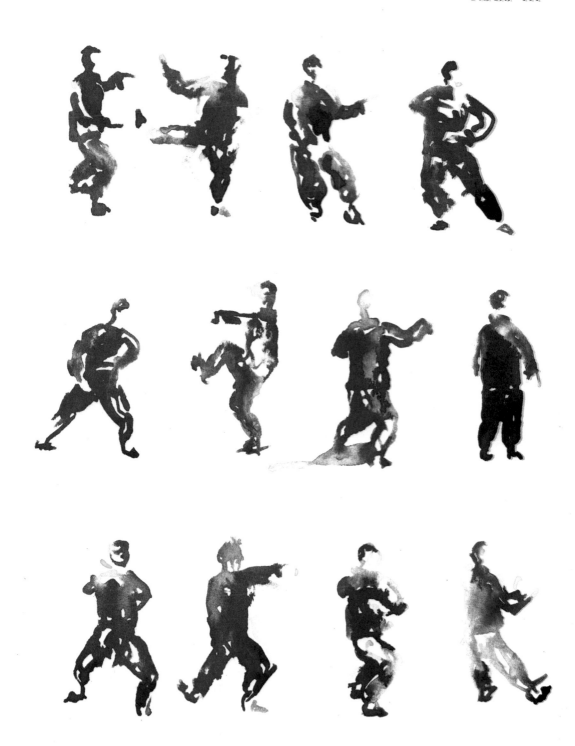

Living with awareness
Eutony

The essence of eutony lies in developing your sensitivity, your ability to observe what is happening in yourself, from the outer boundary of your skin through to the inner space of your bones, joints, and vital organs, and thus to consolidate the roots of your relationship with the outside world.

Developed over the past 45 years by German-born Gerda Alexander, the practice of eutony continues to grow. The word itself derives from the Greek "eu", meaning good or harmonious, and "tonus", meaning tension. Tonus refers to the tension or elasticity of our muscle fibres. It is the first means of communication between baby and mother. All situations in life demand a different level of tonus – for running up stairs, for instance, we need high tonus, for sleep and relaxation, lower tonus. Our emotional life also alters our tonus and the way it is distributed in our bodies. But our tonus – and with it our response to life – can become fixed at one level, inhibiting our movements and preventing us from reacting appropriately to the demands of different situations and experiencing the full range of emotions. The various practices of eutony free your tonus – your movements become more economical, and at the same time more pleasurable. They also have long-lasting effects on your breathing, circulation, and metabolism, and help to balance the autonomic nervous system.

Eutony makes you aware of and helps you to release latent tensions in the body by a process of subtle inner observation. With time, your body sensations become clearer. You begin to realize that your actions, feelings, and thoughts are all rooted in your body. You open up new fields of personal experience, increase your self-knowledge and awareness of others and begin to relate more deeply to the essence of art. Your new body awareness develops into a new awareness as a human being.

Eutony classes follow no pre-established routine, for eutony is not a mechanical technique to be imitated or learned. It is a living, changing process of exploration and, since it contains no set movements or exercises, its principles are easily applied to the activities of everyday life. Closely linked with the arts, eutony frees the path to self-expression and spontaneity. It is of enormous benefit to actors and musicians, as well as to those involved in the visual arts.

As you try the explorations, don't be too eager to feel something immediately, for you may get trapped into imagining rather than truly experiencing a sensation. Simply stay receptive and let the sensations come to you. Work with your eyes open as much as possible, to strengthen your contact with reality. The only real prerequisite for eutony work without a teacher is to allow yourself to discover, through your own authentic sensations, the reality of your body as a source of wisdom and experience.

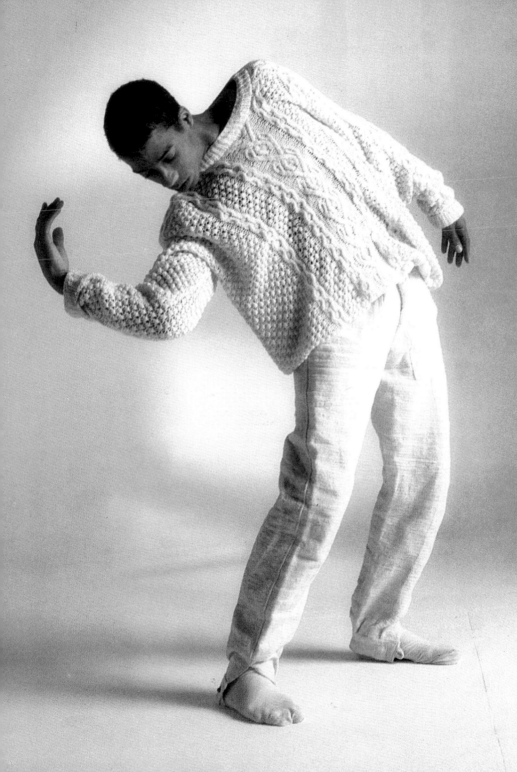

Exploration of touch

Your skin gives you your shape. It is the permeable boundary between yourself and the outside world. Through your skin you give and receive, breathe, perspire, and communicate. Your skin is also your largest organ of information – constantly giving you messages from the environment you live in. Its stimulation is important for the development of the immune, digestive, and breathing systems – if mammals don't lick their newborn, they can die.

By expanding awareness of your skin, you gain a clear sense of your body image. You can develop your perception of this outer boundary by feeling your body touching the support of the floor, or by deliberately touching your body with a bamboo stick. Awakening the sensitivity of your skin may make you yawn or stretch, or cause you to feel a change in temperature or a difference in weight; it may also put you in a special mood. Some people feel weightless when moving with this awareness, or as if they were moving through water, an experience reminiscent of the months spent in the womb.

Without putting this book down, try for a moment to feel your body touching your chair or whatever supports you. Feel where your hand touches the book. Be aware of each finger and thumb. What is the temperature and texture of the book? Does the sensitivity of your fingers vary?

Lie down comfortably on the floor. Feel where you touch its surface with your body – your heels, calves, thighs, and pelvis. Does the floor feel hard or soft? How about your back or *your sides, your neck or your head – can you feel them touching the floor? Can you feel both shoulders, arms and hands against the floor? Which part of your elbows is touching* *the floor? Now try to feel all the parts of your body that touch the floor simultaneously. Be aware of all the nuances of sensation and pressure...*

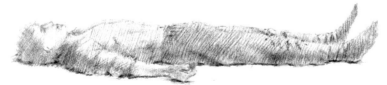

...Now change position. Feel how the pressure and touch change as you slowly move and continue your exploration lying on your front or your *side. Feel the whole envelope of your skin and how it touches your clothes and the air.*

Using a bamboo stick or a pencil, touch the entire skin surface of your right hand and arm. Take your time feeling between your fingers and over your nails, observing any variations in sensitivity between the palm and the back of your hand, the inside and the outside of your arm. Where you can't feel the bamboo, rub a little harder...

...Continue your exploration slowly, passing the bamboo along your armpit and shoulder, and over the right side of your chest and neck. Then lie down on your back and observe the difference in feeling between the left and right sides of your whole body, including the inside of your mouth. Now complete your exploration on the other side.

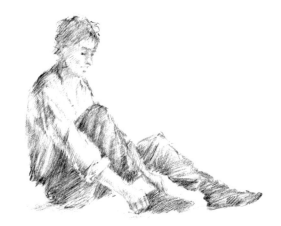

Try for a few days touching just the back of your neck, your hair, and behind your ears, and observe how you feel. Always stay present with the sensation in your skin as you move over your body – never do it mechanically.

You can also develop the sensitivity of your skin in your everyday activities. Feel the water spraying your skin as you shower, or surrounding your body in the bath. Feel your clothes against your skin when you get dressed and be aware of the way your skin moves inside them. As you walk along the street, feel how your body touches your clothes. Are your shoes tight around your feet? Can you feel the air against your skin?

Inner space

We are three-dimensional beings, made of flesh and bone, of tendons and ligaments, of organs, veins, and arteries. All these are part of the "furniture" of our inner space. It is by being in our inner space, learning to feel it as it is, that we can begin to change it – to discover unknown tensions, feel how they are interrelated, and let go of them, freeing our muscles around our bones; to make room inside, opening up in "passages" like the neck, shoulders, and knees; to find and be able to rely on our skeleton; and to equalize our tonus. By becoming aware of our inner substance we can also make contact with our deepest emotions. This contact can ultimately give us access to and allow us to express what is most unique and original about ourselves. When first you begin to explore your inner space, it may feel deserted or lived in, empty or full. Exploring inner space may also make you aware of feeling fragmented. But by your eutony work you can progressively fill and unify your consciousness of inner space and thus improve your contact both with the outer space surrounding you and with other people.

Lie in a comfortable position and try to feel the inside of your mouth, your tongue, your gums, and the space around your teeth. Feel the back of your head on the floor and the way the inner space of your head continues through your neck and into your chest...

...Now start humming and feel how the vibrations from your vocal cords are transmitted throughout your inner space, through your bones, joints, and organs, down to the soles of your feet.

On another day, put 1 hand on each side of your pelvis and try to get a clear feeling of the distance between them – from the back of 1 hand through the palm touching the pelvis to the

palm and back of the other hand, and vice versa...

...Then put 1 hand on your lower belly and feel the distance through to the back of the pelvis, and vice versa...

...Now try to feel your inner space continuing down from the pelvis into your right leg and foot. Then, without closing your inner space, roll your heel gently against the floor. See how far up your body you can feel this movement.

Vital stretch

Look at a cat when it wakes up from sleep or finishes a meal. It will move part of its body, pause, perhaps yawn, then move another part, until the whole body appears to be moved from within. Babies do just the same, if left to wake up in their own rhythm. This spontaneous stretching is one of the most primitive and fundamental ways of equalizing tonus and of being present. It can also lead to deep yawns – themselves an expression of an inner stretch. In itself, it is not a voluntary movement, but a spontaneous response to an inner impulse. You can provide the initial stimulus by slightly shifting your position or by rubbing or stretching yourself against a firm surface. Then simply allow the movements to happen, without directing them, noticing the sequence of sensations in your whole being. The impulse to move may be very slight or may increase unexpectedly, and it will vary from day to day. Good times to explore this vital stretch are when you wake up, after a long time in one position, or before, after, or even during any of the other eutonic practices described in this chapter.

Without putting down the book or changing position, begin to observe the sensations in your body. Feel if there is any discomfort, any need to move. If there is not, simply wait. When there is, surrender to the need, observing how you feel as you move...

...See if you can let the movement extend through your whole body, if you can let yourself "be stretched". To allow the movement through, you may need to let go in your skin, release your joints, allow space between your ribs, or release in your stomach...

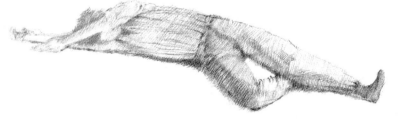

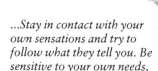

...Stay in contact with your own sensations and try to follow what they tell you. Be sensitive to your own needs,

exploring whatever movements feel pleasurable and involve the totality of your body. Don't hurry.

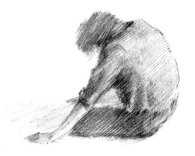

Exploration of contact

In making eutonic "contact", we consciously feel beyond the limits of our skin. Being in contact with objects or people means going toward them and remaining open to them in true communication. It helps to break down the barriers of isolation. Contact is a phenomenon that exists normally at an unconscious level but you can consciously reinforce it, as shown here. Making contact consciously harmonizes tonus and breathing and increases the circulation. Some concrete examples help to clarify the concept: a blind person makes contact with the ground through his stick; a driver parking his car extends his body right to the left-hand back corner of his vehicle; and a good actress will reach a member of the audience sitting right at the back of the stalls with the strength of her contact. Difficulties with making contact may be a sign that you don't like what you are doing, that you reject something – a typist who does not like her work or her typewriter, for example, may cut the free flow through her fingers into the keys, and get cramps or headaches as a result.

Sit comfortably on a chair, holding an apple in 1 hand. Feel your palm and each of your fingers touching the skin of the apple and notice what information you can pick up about it through your hand. Now feel beyond the part of the apple you are touching, completing its full shape with your awareness. Feel its roundness and weight, and feel into its flesh, through to the core....

...Be aware, also, of the relationship between your hand and the apple, observing how it helps you to feel your hand's fleshy and bony parts. Can you still feel the boundary between your hand and the apple?

Feel into the chair too – the seat and the 4 legs, all supported by the floor. And through the chair, as well as with your feet, feel the thickness of the floor and how it is there, carrying you, all the time. Now put the apple down. Compare the left side of your body to the right.

Try this with other objects too. If you play a musical instrument, try to make this contact with it and observe how both the sound of the instrument and your own well-being improve.

Drawing movements

Stretching from one part of your body, then allowing this stretch to develop into "drawings" in space is an excellent way of exploring an entirely new range of movements. It frees you to move lightly and spontaneously, just as you do when, in daily life for example, someone offers you something you like to eat, and your hand moves toward it effortlessly, without your even thinking about it. Try it now. Lying down on the floor, begin stretching from one heel across your other leg, letting your whole body follow. Feel when your pelvis starts following, when each of your vertebrae becomes engaged in the movement, your waist, your chest....Keep your shoulders and arms relaxed and allow your head to roll passively on the floor.

Lie on your back, choose a point on the ceiling, and reach toward it with your hand, allowing your whole body to follow. Try this again, reaching toward different points in the room with other parts of the body.

Standing upright now, feel your right elbow, touching it if necessary. Then start exploring the whole space in front of you, behind, above, and below you, letting yourself be led by the elbow. If you had a paint brush attached to your elbow, the result of your movement would be a huge 3-dimensional drawing.

Now, lying down again, observe the feeling in your whole body, noticing any differences between your left and right sides.

Exploration of pushing

In eutonic pushing, or "repousser", you use the resistance of the floor as a support into which you direct a force – either to move yourself, to change position, or to move an object. You somehow take the force from the floor and allow it to be transmitted through your bone structure. Your body is transparent to the force, your inner space is open, your muscles are free. There is no superfluous expenditure of energy, no feeling of effort or tiredness. Your breathing stays free. Pushing raises your tonus and stimulates your awareness of your bones. After trying the exploration, observe how you feel and what mood you are in, compared to your feelings after a session working with your skin or with inner space.

Lie down on your back and feel your contact with the floor. Become aware of the way the floor supports your right elbow, then push with your elbow straight down into the floor. Observe which part of your body is lifted up. Try pushing with your elbow into the floor at different angles, taking note of the effect on other parts of the body.

Now try pushing down into the floor with your head, your sacrum, or one heel. Notice which part of your body lifts up.

Lie on your back and bend one leg. With your foot, push into the floor at a 45-degree angle, observing how it affects the rest of your body, especially your spine. (This is very good for backache). Release in your buttocks, back, stomach, and *thigh muscles, while allowing the force of the pushing to go through your bones. Continue to explore, pushing with 1 or both feet at different angles into the floor. You may find the pushing turns your body completely over.*

Exploration of bones

We often forget we have bones, even though the framework they provide supports and protects the entire body. Getting in touch with your bones – and knowing you can rely on their support – has a powerful effect on your whole being. It gives you a sense of inner security and stability which allows you to let go of superfluous muscle tension. Although these tensions may have served to protect you, they have also served to limit your sensitivity, movement, and expression. Feeling your bones, their individual shape and quality, their functions and movements may lead to surprising discoveries. The sensation of bone is not necessarily one of numbness or density, but often one of lightness, porousness, and clarity.

In exploring the bones of your foot, as shown here, it's important to remain open to what you may find, without any expectations or preconceived images. For this reason, we have not included an anatomical drawing of the bones, but suggest you consult an anatomy book after doing the explorations.

Explore the bones of your right foot with your hands. Discover how many bones you have in each toe, and how far inside your feet the bones of the toes reach. Test the mobility of each joint. Initially you can use your hands to mobilize your bones, but after a while, try to focus your attention on each bone in turn, letting the bone itself direct the movement. Don't expect anything spectacular. The intention to move 1 bone at a time is more important than whether or not it visibly moves...

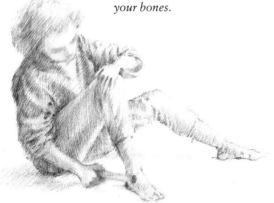

You can also knock on your bones with a bamboo stick and feel the bone structure transmitting the vibrations. By knocking on your ankle bones you can realize the shape and structure of your tibia and fibula. Try to receive the vibrations at the other end of your bones.

Before exploring your right foot lie down and observe the effect of what you have done on the whole body. Is there a difference between the left and right sides of your face or are they balanced? Stand up and take a few steps, walking with the feeling of your bone structure carrying you.

Transport and posture

Our posture, movements, and attitudes are all an expression of ourselves; they are part of ourselves and can't just be dismissed. In eutony there's no such thing as "bad" posture or "wrong" movement. Eutony is never taught by imitation – each of us must find for ourselves the posture most appropriate for our individual structure. Posture is aligned through working with transport, the conscious use of the "postural reflex". This reflex is the primary reflex that babies are born with and which they use later on when they learn to stand. Transport is the anti-gravity force triggered by your weight on your feet. It goes up through your skeleton and liberates the entire peripheral musculature. This difficult concept becomes clearer as your tonus is balanced through other eutonic practices. To let the transport go through, you need the resistance of a support to give you in return the sense of your own inner structure.

Finding your hip joints
Many of us harbour misguided images of our bodies and these images restrict our posture and the way we move. Discovering where certain strategic joints are situated in your body or which bones are connected to one another can make an amazing difference to the way you stand and move. Stand up and put your hands over your hip joints. Are they at the side of your body, as shown below, or in front, as shown below left...?

...Bend 1 knee and lift it up, then draw with it in the air. Move your pelvis. Now can you feel where the joint is between thigh bone and pelvis? Take a look at the skeleton...and correct the position of your fingers. Many of us mistake the rounded, protruding ends of our thigh bones, known as the trochanters, for our hip joints.

As a result, instead of the pelvis being carried upward by the hip joints, it falls down between the trochanters, resulting in circulatory and digestive problems, and progressive degeneration of the hip joints. Finding how close to each other your hip joints are helps you to find your transport.

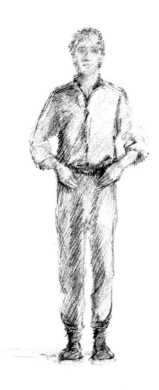
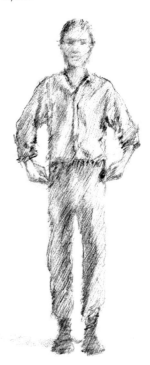

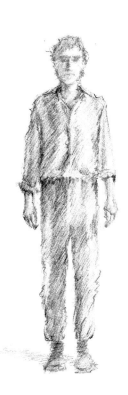

Finding transport

Stand with your feet parallel, the same width apart as your hip joints. Push down vertically with your first metatarsal bones, feeling how your whole body lifts up. Follow the passage of the transport up – through the arch of your feet, through the tibias, knee joints, and femurs, the hip joints, to the small pelvic girdle, where the two forces from the feet meet, up through the sacrum and bodies of the spinal vertebrae to the uppermost vertebra, the atlas, and on up to the top of your head. Now distribute your weight evenly between your heels and your first metatarsals. Then try also walking with transport, endeavouring to entrust your weight to your bones.

"At first, I could never feel anything in the classes. Then suddenly I realized that the feelings had been there all the time. But it is all so subtle – feelings are so subtle."

"...After two years of sessions, eutony has changed radically the way I use and think about my body...I have acquired new ways to be in my body, ways that feel easily natural to me, unforced, like an inherent order that I have had revealed to me."

Quotes from Eutony students

Skeleton and bone

In many cultures, unlike ours, bones are associated with life – with strength, solidity, reality, actuality, independence, and essence. In Turkey, for example, relatives are said to be of the same bone, rather than of the same blood. In fact bone is far from dead. It is a living material, capable of response and change and constantly regenerated throughout our lifetime. It is, after all, in the bone marrow that our red and white blood cells are manufactured. Its inner structure is an amazing piece of architecture, beautifully demonstrating the laws of force.

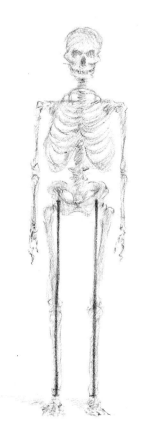

Expanding sensation
Kum Nye

Kum Nye is a system of gentle meditative self-healing exercises which help you to get in touch with yourself, stripping away layers of conditioning locked in the body and enhancing your appreciation of life. Brought to the West and systematized by Tarthang Tulku Rinpoche, it originates from Tibet, where, as a process of self-exploration, it formed part of both the medical and spiritual traditions of Tibetan Buddhism.

In Kum Nye (pronounced Koom Nyay), health and disease are considered in terms of energy and feeling. When feelings are blocked, and body and mind are out of contact, the free flow of energy is constricted, lowering vitality and laying us open to physical or mental illness. In a state of health, our energy flows smoothly and we are in touch with our feelings, integrating body and mind. The key to a balanced relationship with ourselves and the world around us lies in contacting and being aware of our feelings. The basic process of Kum Nye therefore consists of stimulating and expanding feelings and sensations.

But in order to experience and integrate your feelings fully, relaxation is essential. When you are totally relaxed, your sensitivity increases and you can open up to new dimensions of feeling and sensation which unite physical and mental awareness. Your mind becomes clear and open, your body alive and dynamic. As you practise the exercises of Kum Nye, the quality of your relaxation deepens. At first you are mainly aware of releasing sensations of physical tension and pain, but as these gradually dissolve, you reach further into the exercises, letting go of emotional and mental holding patterns that lie deeper. Your senses awaken, heightening your perception of colour, sound, taste, and so on. Ultimately you transcend the ego, experiencing only a joyful melting quality that suffuses your whole being.

Gentle self-healing exercises make up the main practice of Kum Nye, most performed in very slow motion and followed by a period of sitting still and relaxing. Accompanied by awareness and breathing techniques, the exercises encourage a quality of deep stillness which allows you to become conscious of and expand sensations and emotions of which you are normally unaware. Each exercise affects particular parts of the body, stimulating specific qualities of feeling and releasing both physical and psychological tension. The feelings and sensations aroused soothe and massage the body from inside – in fact the literal meaning of Kum Nye is "inner massage" or massage of the higher or "subtle" body. Other Kum Nye practices include self-massage, meditation using mantras, and working more specifically with the body's *chakras* or energy centres.

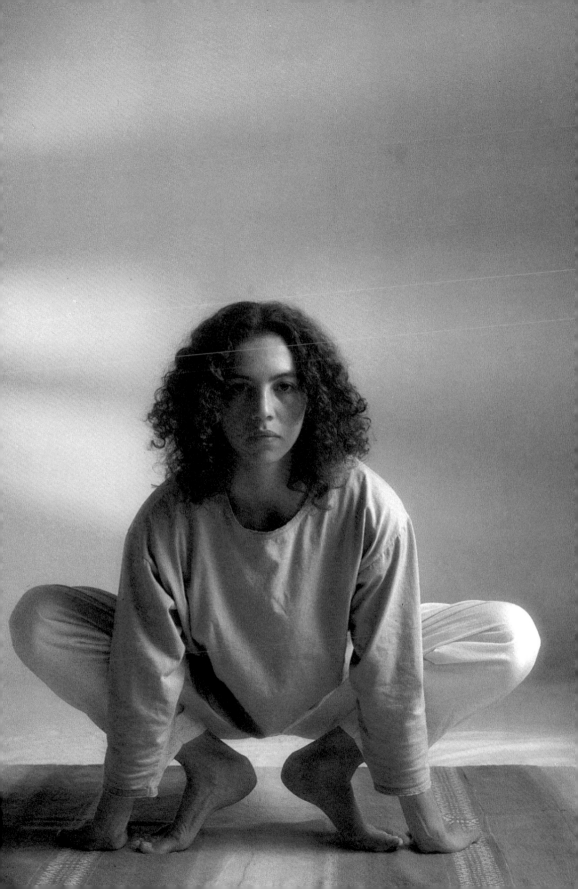

Foundations of practice

In essence Kum Nye is about learning to be aware of and to expand feelings and sensations. But to enjoy the full benefits of the exercises, there are a number of principles you need to understand. Firstly, any movement you make in an exercise should be extremely slow – so slow that from outside it may be barely perceptible. This deliberate slowness increases the quality of awareness and is essential if you are to be open to the nuances of sensation and feeling stimulated by the exercise. Secondly, you should approach each exercise openly, without expectation – simply be mindful of your feelings, without labelling or analysing them. Perform each movement with relaxed concentration, but don't try too hard or be too eager to get results, as this will prevent you from opening to the immediacy of your own experience. Start by practising just one of the exercises for a few weeks, then add others one by one. After each exercise it's important to spend five to ten minutes sitting quietly and using balanced breathing, in order to allow the sensations aroused by the exercise to continue internally.

Practical matters
Your external surroundings reflect and influence your state of mind, so try to do Kum Nye in a calm, harmonious environment. Ideally, practise in the morning, before or at least an hour after eating. Take off your shoes, and wear loose clothing that won't inhibit free movement or interfere with the sensations engendered by the exercises.

Sitting
There are 7 "gestures" or details to be observed in the sitting position, which assist the flow of energy in the body:

1. Sit cross-legged, with your buttocks on a cushion so that your pelvis is higher than your legs. Or sit on an upright chair, feet flat on the floor.

2. Place your hands, palms down, on your knees. Relax your shoulders, arms, and hands.

3. Find a balanced position for your spine – keep it straight but relaxed, so that energy can flow easily up from your lower body.

4. Draw your neck back a little and stretch it slightly upward.

5. Keep your eyes half-open, and your gaze "soft", looking down the ridge of your nose, toward the ground.

6. Have your mouth slightly open and relax your jaw.

7. Rest the tip of your tongue on your palate, just behind your front teeth.

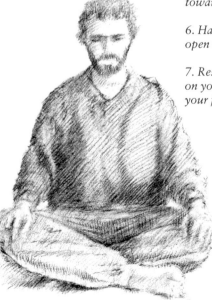

Balanced breathing
Both during all Kum Nye
exercises and in the period of
sitting quietly afterward, you
use "balanced breathing". This
means breathing evenly and
slowly through the nose and
the mouth at the same time,
with the mouth slightly open,
and the tongue curled to touch
the palate. Exhalation and
inhalation should be so soft
and subtle that you are hardly
aware of them.

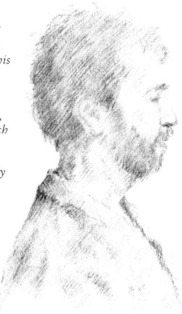

Breathing in this way relaxes
the throat centre and allows
the energy to reach both head
and heart chakras (see p.57).
Practise simply sitting and
breathing until you get used to
it. After a while, you will begin
to notice the vitality it brings.

Expanding sensation
While practising Kum Nye,
many sensations will arise,
both physical and emotional,
powerful and more subtle. As
soon as you begin an exercise,
become aware of any feelings
or sensations that are
awakened. Stimulating and
expanding these sensations or
feeling tones is fundamental to
Kum Nye. While sitting quietly
after doing the exercises, stay
with the sensations and allow
them to continue, softening
around them. Following them
with your awareness, let them
expand and spread throughout
your body, and even beyond.
You can expand even the most
subtle sensations in this way.

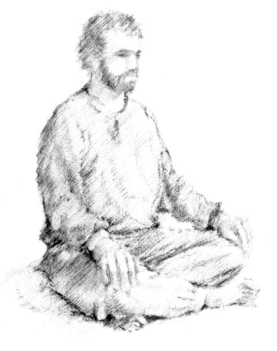

Melting tension

It is hard to relax your body if your mind is tense or preoccupied – tension or stiffness in the body is always linked to mental or emotional restlessness or unease. As you practise this exercise, don't *try* to relax. Simply observe what you are thinking about or feeling, without dwelling on it or analysing it. Stillness will come by itself. Keep your awareness in your pelvis and hip joints and take note of any movement of energy up the spine. Notice if one side of your body feels stiffer than the other and see if this imbalance is the same or different next time you come to do the exercise. As your resistance gradually melts, you will discover that you can lift your knee a little higher.

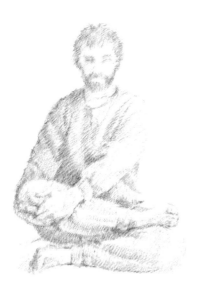 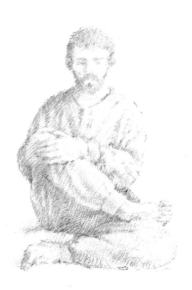

Melting tension
Sit down and cross your legs, resting your right ankle on your left thigh. Interlock your fingers and clasp them around your right knee. Then, keeping your back straight, very slowly pull your knee up a little way. Hold the position when you feel any resistance and allow it to melt...

...When it releases, pull your knee up a little further. Then slowly lower it down again, following the sensations in your whole body. Practise this 3 or 9 times, moving more slowly each time. Repeat the exercise the same number of times on the other side.

Now sit for 5-10 minutes, and practise balanced breathing, following and expanding the sensations engendered by the exercise (see pp.126-7).

Loosening up

In Loosening up, you work on letting go of tension in your upper back, neck, shoulders and chest, as well as in your hips. As with all Kum Nye exercises, however, the process works at a mental and emotional level and not just physically. While doing the exercise, make sure that you don't turn your head when you turn your shoulders – keep it facing forward throughout. And use your breathing to monitor how you are. Stopping breathing is a way of holding back feeling – so if you find you are holding your breath try to observe when, and what you are unwilling to feel. If strong feelings come up, bring them into balanced breathing.

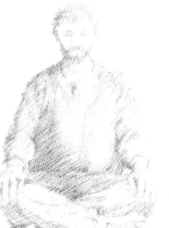

Loosening up
Sit cross-legged, with your hands over your knees, arms and back straight. Moving as slowly as possible, twist your upper body to the left, so that your right shoulder points forward and your left shoulder back. Allow your left hand to slide up over your thigh, bending your arm, but keep the right arm straight. Then, equally slowly, reverse the position.

Do this 3 or 9 times, then spend 5-10 minutes in the sitting posture, following and expanding the sensations (pp.126-7).

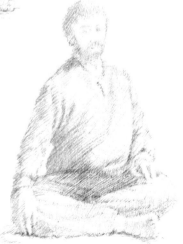

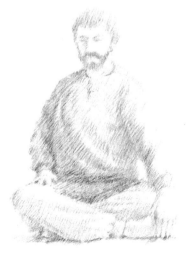

Touching time

In practising Kum Nye, you use your breathing to dissolve tension. Each time you encounter a point of resistance in an exercise, simply bring your breath to meet it while you hold the position. Breathe with the pain and tension, then slowly exhale and relax the area. It's important that you meet any feelings of resistance in the body gently, softening or melting the boundaries around the pain or stiffness. The thighs and back muscles are stretched in Touching time, and energy that has been held in the hips and lower back is released. If you find it too painful to maintain the position when you bend forward, simply straighten up again slowly.

Touching time
Sit with the soles of your feet together, knees out to the side. Pull your feet in to the body as close as possible. Place your hands on your knees and press down. Keep your shoulders level. Now, very slowly, lean as far forward as you can, moving from the hips, without rounding your back. Stay down for 1-3 minutes, focusing your awareness in your pelvis or at the base of your spine...

Relax your belly and breathe softly through your nose and mouth. Then come up again, slowly straightening your back. Sit for a few moments before repeating the exercise a couple more times. Then, when you have finished, sit for 5 to 10 minutes, allowing the sensations aroused by the exercise to expand (see pp.126-7).

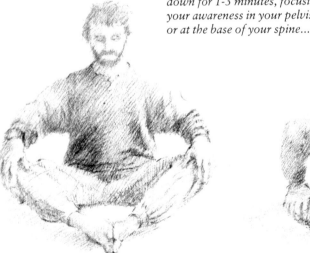

Sensing energy

This exercise is in two parts. In the first, you move your outstretched arms forward and back using your shoulders to direct the movement. In the second, you bend your arms up then lower them again, moving only your forearms while keeping your upper arms still. As you perform these slow repetitive sequences, let your full awareness dwell on your experience in the movement, so that body and mind act as one. Whenever you meet a sense of resistance, pause and allow it to release, then see if you can go further. Observe any feelings stimulated at your heart *chakra*, the energy centre in the middle of your chest, during the second part of the exercise.

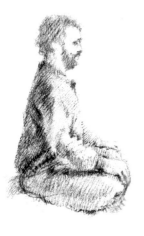 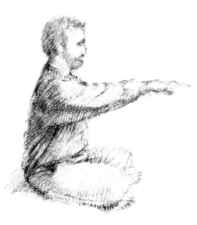 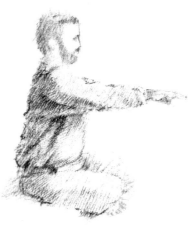

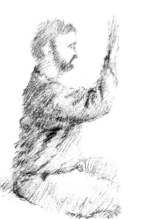

Sensing energy
Sit cross-legged, with your hands on your knees. Slowly raise your arms up to shoulder level and stretch forward with your hands, palms down. Now pull your shoulders back very slowly, then once again reach your hands forward. Repeat this sequence 9 times, moving only your shoulders and arms, keeping the rest of your body still...

...Then bring your hands down to your knees and, with your shoulders in a neutral position, sit quietly. After a few minutes, raise your arms again and bend your elbows until your hands are pointing up to the ceiling, then slowly bring your hands down. Do this movement 9 times, then sit still for 5-10 minutes (as on pp.126-7).

Energizing body and mind

The exercises of Kum Nye are very different from other forms of physical exercise. Although they stretch and strengthen the body, improving physical health, this is not their sole aim. They are primarily designed to stimulate feelings and internal energies and thus enhance functioning at all levels of being – physical, mental, and emotional. Each exercise is geared to a particular effect, working on releasing specific sensations and energies. In Energizing body and mind, you may experience a sensation of opening in the belly or lower back and heat between the shoulder-blades. You may also find that your breathing changes or your legs and pelvis tremble. It is important that you don't strain to hold the position – the essence of Kum Nye is relaxation.

Energizing body and mind
Lie on your back with your arms outstretched, palms up. Then bend your knees, bring your feet together, and let your knees drop open to the side, keeping your soles on the floor...

...Now raise your pelvis as high as possible off the floor, supporting your weight on your feet and shoulders. Stay in this position for a couple of minutes, then slowly lower your hips down again, straighten each leg in turn and rest, arms by your sides.

Do this 2 more times, then bring your knees in toward your chest, and rest your hands on them. Remain in this position for 5-10 minutes (instead of sitting), immersing yourself in the sensations that you have stimulated.

Flying

As its name suggests, Flying describes a smooth, even movement which, when done properly, makes you feel light and free. You need to move your arms up and down extremely slowly, taking either a minute or two minutes to go in each direction. Don't be tempted to speed up the movement. The exercise stimulates energy at the heart *chakra*, the energy centre in the middle of the chest, and may cause a feeling of heat around your arms and hands. It also quietens and clears the mind, freeing you from restless thoughts and anxiety.

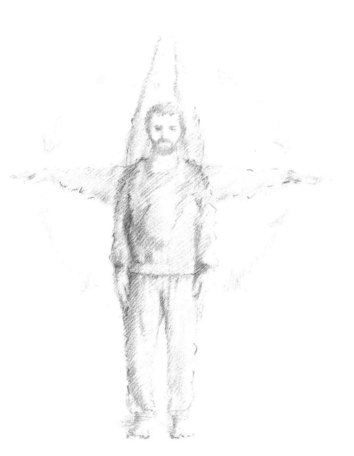

Flying
Stand with your weight evenly distributed on both legs and your feet comfortably apart, arms by your sides. Very slowly lift your arms straight out to the sides and up above your head, until the backs of your hands are practically touching. Close your eyes and relax your body while you hold the position for a few minutes, experiencing the movement of energy...

...Then very slowly separate your arms and, moving them at an even pace, bring them down by your sides. When you repeat this flying movement, stretch up a little with your arms when they are overhead. Practise the complete movement 9 times altogether. Finish by sitting quietly for 5-10 minutes (as on pp.126-7).

Interacting body and mind

In Kum Nye, the integration and balance of body and mind are considered of supreme importance. But in order for this integration to be possible, a certain relaxation is necessary, and at times you may be too tense or agitated, mentally or physically, to contact your feelings well during an exercise. If this happens, it's a good idea to spend a little time relaxing in the sitting posture before you start, practising balanced breathing and simply sensing each part of the body, from head to feet, allowing any tension to soften and melt. In Interacting body and mind you release tension in the arms, shoulders, back, and legs. Don't strain as you practise the exercise, and keep breathing softly and evenly throughout.

Interacting body and mind
Stand with your feet a few inches apart and your arms by your sides. Point your left foot to the left and put your right foot about 12 inches in front of it, pointing forward, with your 2 heels in line. Slowly raise

your arms straight out to the sides and up to shoulder height, then bend them and put your hands on your shoulders, with your thumbs behind and your fingers in front. Press your hands down...

...Now very slowly turn your torso as far as possible to the left, leading with your left elbow, and bend forward. Still with your head down, without pausing, continue turning to the right, then come up straight again, looking up at

the ceiling as you do so. Do this 3 or 9 times, then reverse the position of your feet and repeat the movement, this time rotating first to the right. End by sitting quietly for 5-10 minutes (see pp.126-7).

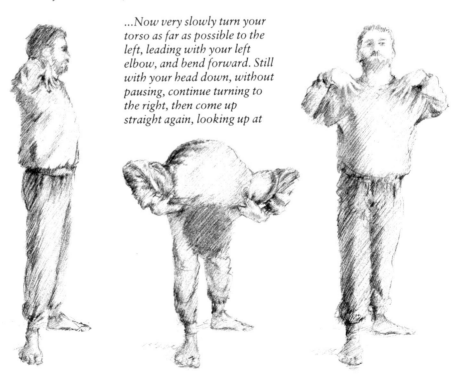

Relieving negativity

Since your emotions are so intimately linked with your body, it's possible to release and transform them through a physical posture. Relieving negativity releases energy in both the legs and chest and allows you to let go of any destructive or limiting emotions. If you find the exercise painful, simply try to soften around the area of pain or tension and rest your awareness on the sensation rather than the thought of pain. This will enable you to release and make use of the energy that has been locked in tension and extend how long you can hold the position. While you practise the exercise you may feel energy moving in your legs and at the base of your spine.

Relieving negativity
Stand with your feet apart, arms by your sides. Then put your hands on your sides, as near as possible to your armpits, fingers pointing down. Try not to hunch your shoulders. Now bend your legs, as if sitting down, until *you reach a special place where you will sense a difference in energy. Now look up at the ceiling and stay in this position for up to a minute. Then slowly stand up straight again and, without pausing, bend forward from the waist so that your upper body is parallel to the floor. Pause here briefly then, once again, slowly bend your legs until you come to the special point of energy. When your legs start to tremble, hold the position for up to a minute,* *breathing gently. Then gradually straighten your legs and bring your torso up, allowing your arms to hang once more by your sides. Rest for a few minutes, either standing or sitting, then do it twice more. Sit for 5-10 minutes afterward, letting the feelings continue (see pp.126-7).*

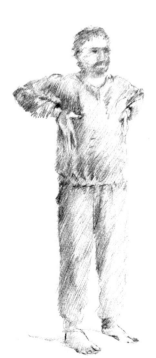

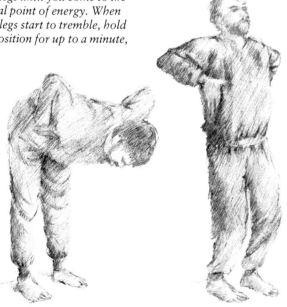

Running free

Body awareness need not be a matter of moving slowly, as in T'ai chi or Kum Nye. It can also be gained in more dynamic forms of exercise, such as running, swimming, cycling, or skiing, provided they are approached with the right attitude. The secret is to regard the exercise you choose as a means to explore your body's capabilities and deepen your relationship with yourself, not as a way to test or discipline yourself. Essentially, it means being gentle with yourself, moving always without strain and without a feeling of competitiveness, and using the time you exercise for pleasure, not as an endurance test to see how fast or how far you can go.

Running is a great way of getting in tune with your body. It is more than just a sport. It's a form of meditation, a way of self-discovery. When you run, you move inside yourself to find peace and stillness. You experience the earth beneath your feet, and your connection to it. You can use visualization to gain more control of the physical and mental process of running and broaden your horizons. You can run any distance and speed that feel right for you.

Taking the first step toward "getting in shape" is the hardest, but it is possible to remain in touch with your good intentions. By letting your body determine the type, speed, frequency, and duration of running, and dropping any expectations from the outset of "how it should be done", you can discover the part inside you that longs to run. Healthwise, running regularly has many physical rewards – weight loss, increased strength and muscle tone, a stronger heart, better circulation, a clearer skin, and sounder sleep. Its mental, spiritual, and emotional benefits are just as numerous. Of course, it can be hard work. But mostly it's fun, a game to be enjoyed. For basically, our bodies love to move, to dance, to fly over the earth and, through running, you can discover the joy that is innate in all of us as living, moving human beings.

In this chapter you will find advice on how to make running your own. The focus is on getting you started in a way that works for you, on preventing injury, and on creating an internal environment and attitude which will carry you into a future of enjoyable running. As you continue reading, imagine yourself, dressed and ready to run, doing the warm-up exercises, then running outside and experimenting with your breath, with visualization, and with grounding. Imagine how you'll feel at the end of your first run – feel the pounding heart, the heated limbs, the sweating skin. Allow yourself to go through all of the fears and excuses as to why it won't work for you. Then, after airing all your resistances, re-read the chapter, imagining once again doing the warm-ups, the run, and the cool-down. Stay in touch with the knowledge that you create your own experience.

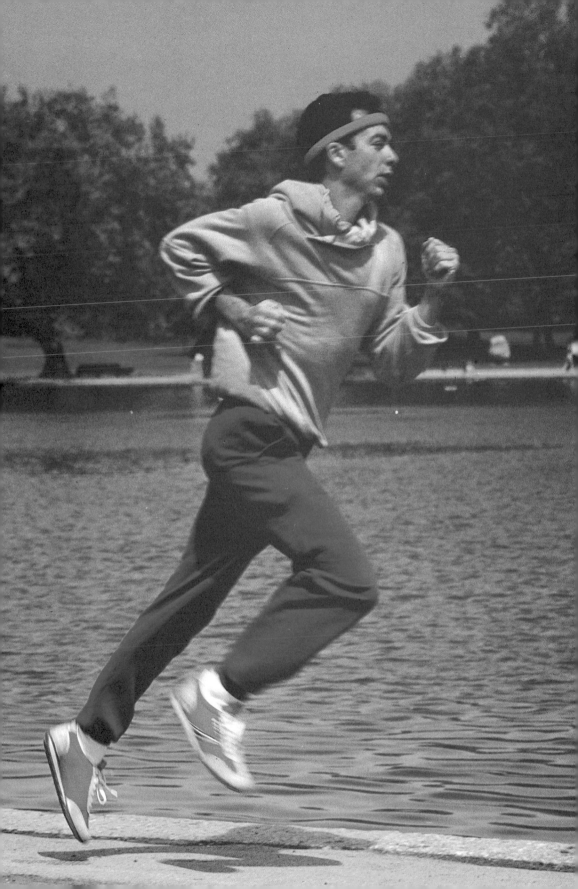

Before you start

While running, jogging, and walking are ways of increasing body awareness, they are also sports, and you need to prepare yourself properly. Check with your doctor if you have any doubts about the advisability of running for you. If you do have a question about your fitness, follow this chapter through, but substitute *walking* each time you see *running*. In fact, walking is how we begin, anyway. For the first few weeks, try doing the warm-ups, going for a short, brisk walk, and then doing the cool-down exercises. Gradually, as the walking becomes easier, start to add in short jogs, alternating between walking and running for short intervals. At this point you might walk, with short running spurts, for 15 minutes. Slowly begin to decrease the amount of time you spend walking until you are running the entire time. Always make sure to leave yourself enough time to get dressed, warm up, run/walk, cool down, and take a shower. If you want to see a real improvement in your fitness, you need to run at least three times each week. Three to five times is ideal for health benefits, but always take at least one day off a week.

Clothing and equipment
A good pair of running shoes is all you need to start running — they can make the difference between enjoyment and misery.

Find a sporting goods store where you feel comfortable trying on lots of pairs of shoes and asking lots of questions. Wear the socks you are going to run in to try on the shoes. Take time to do your research and buy the best, most comfortable shoes you can afford.

Wear loose, comfortable clothing for running, and don't overdress. Wear something to protect you in windy, rainy, or cold weather. Cover your head in winter to keep warm and in summer to protect against the sun. And always use cotton or wool socks with no wrinkles — they cause blisters.

Warming up

Warming up should be considered an integral part of your run – it is essential to prevent injury. Spend a full ten minutes warming up each time you run. This is time for stretching and increasing the blood supply to the muscles; for creating a break from whatever you were doing before; and for mentally and emotionally getting into the right mood for the run. As you do the stretching exercises that follow, allow your mind and emotions to become equal partners with your body. Be aware of how you feel about warming up and running today. If you experience any negative or unhelpful attitudes, just mentally step back and watch yourself feeling them. Then remember the enthusiasm and interest you felt when you first decided to run. Think of a time when you had a particularly wonderful feeling during or after a run or exercise session. Everyone loses their inspiration at times, and we all have lazy days. On days when you have planned a run but just aren't in the mood, consciously ask yourself: do I want to go with my current feeling, or with my original intention to run? After you decide, make the most of whichever you end up doing!

Warm-up guidelines

Do:
- *Breathe regularly and deeply.*
- *Allow gravity to do the work.*
- *Relax your face, shoulders and stomach.*
- *Go at your own pace.*
- *Sink into stretches, for a full 30 seconds if possible.*
- *Release as many muscles as possible.*
- *Modify stretches so they work for you.*
- *Have patience with yourself.*

Don't:
- *Bounce.*
- *Hold your breath.*
- *Work at it.*
- *Stretch to the point of pain.*
- *Expect to touch your toes tomorrow.*
- *Grit your teeth.*
- *Tense up.*

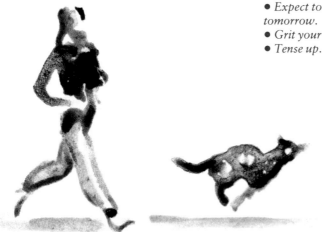

Times and repetitions (reps)
given are approximate, to be
used as guidelines only. Do
what feels best for you.

Relaxation
(3 mins)
Sit comfortably or lie on your
back, and close your eyes.
Keep still, watching your
breath and surrendering to
gravity. Allow yourself to find
a still point or centre inside,
and breathe in and out of that
place for 3 minutes.

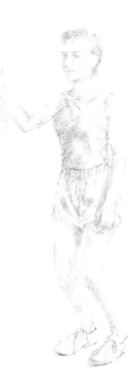

Ankle and foot stretch
(1 min, 5 reps)
Stand with your feet hip-width
apart. Gently bend your knees
until you feel a pull in the
ankles and calves (as shown
left). After a count of 5, slowly
straighten your knees. Keeping
the legs straight, slowly raise
the heels until you are standing
on your toes. Spread the toes
out like tree roots, and relax
into the position for a count of
5. Then slowly return your
heels to the ground.

Calf and hamstring stretch
(2 mins, 2 reps each leg)
Stand about 1 foot from a wall,
placing both hands at chest-
height against it. Move your
right foot back and bend your
left knee, keeping your back
leg straight. Count to 30. Vary
the stretch by leaning into the
wall, changing the distance
between your feet, moving
your pelvis forward and
pushing your back heel more
firmly into the ground. Repeat,
bending the right knee.

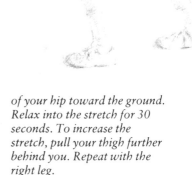

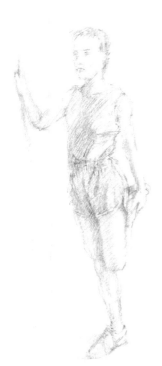

Thigh stretch
(2 mins, 2 reps each leg)
Standing on your right leg,
raise your left foot up behind
you and grab it with your left
hand (see left). Gently pull the
foot toward your buttocks.
Imagine the leg dropping out

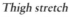

of your hip toward the ground.
Relax into the stretch for 30
seconds. To increase the
stretch, pull your thigh further
behind you. Repeat with the
right leg.

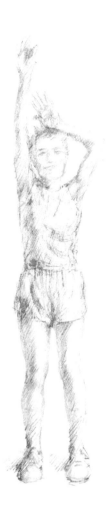

Dorsal stretch

(2 mins, 2 reps)
Standing with your feet
shoulder-width apart, inhale
and raise both arms. Exhale
and stretch your right arm as
high as you can, stretching the
whole right side. Inhale and
stretch the left arm and side
upward. Repeat once more
with each arm. Then exhale,
lower your arms, and let your
shoulders drop.

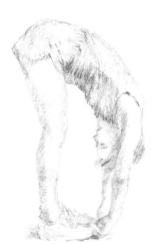

Bending your knees very
slightly, allow your head to
drop to your chest, and slowly
roll down until you are
hanging in a rag-doll position.
Hang like this for 30 seconds,
then bend your knees further,
and roll up gently, with your
head coming up last.
Straighten your legs.

Abdominal and lower back strengthener

(1 min, 3-10 reps)
Lie on your back with your
knees bent, feet flat. Exhale
and push your lower back into
the ground. Inhale and cross
your arms over your chest.
Exhale, pull your stomach in,
and sit up halfway. Then
inhale and lower your body to
*the floor, **keeping your lower***
back pressed to the ground.
Relax, then repeat.

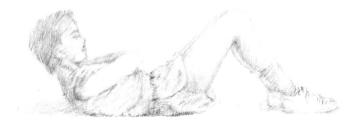

The Run

"Jogging" often conjures up visions of incredible tedium, but there's no need for this. To make your run more enjoyable, there are numerous aspects you can vary. Varying the speed you run not only gives you more control, it also brings greater health benefits. Try starting out with a brisk walk, then shifting into a loose bouncing run, shaking your shoulders and legs. You may then want to jog for a spell, to warm up, with occasional sprints at different speeds for interest. Slow down to a brisk walk whenever you need to rest.

Finding your own rhythm

New runners often become stiff out of self-consciousness, or, without realizing it, try to imitate other runners they've seen. But if you look closely, you'll notice that every runner you see uses a different style, a different gait. Watch children and animals run. Then go out to an open field, forget anything you ever thought or felt about running, and run. Move fast, skip, prance, go forward and backward and in circles. Run for the joy of moving your body, as a child, or a gazelle, or a jaguar would. Experiment with various length strides and ways of using your arms as you shift gaits. Varying gait and arm use as you become stronger and more accustomed to running heightens the interest of your runs considerably.

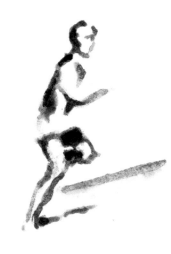

Varying terrain and time of day

Plan several routes that differ in terms of distance, area, surroundings, and terrain. You may want to have a short run which has a slight uphill climb in it, and a slightly longer one with more downslope. Have at least one route on packed earth or grass, and, if possible, try at times to run on a beach, barefoot. You may run better at one time of day, but feel better after a run at a different time. Try running at a few different times of day before you settle on the one best for you. Bear in mind that routes, too, will differ according to the time of day.

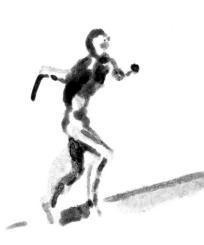

Grounding, breathing, and meditation

Running is a great way to experience your groundedness, to actually be in the lower half of your body, aware of your connection to the earth. Feel the impact of each footfall moving up through your legs, pelvis, and lower back. Concentrate on feeling the different surfaces that you run on. Try visualizing your pelvis and hip sockets as you move. Use your breathing as a feed-back mechanism. Before you even start running, make sure you can breathe abdominally and walk at the same time. If you do get out of breath when you run, you're going too fast or for too long. Allow your exhalation to be longer than your inhalation, creating a rhythm. For example, inhale for two steps and exhale for three. An effective meditation you can use while running is to count each breath after you exhale, counting until you get to five breaths, and then starting with one again. Focusing on a part of your body can also become a meditation: on your feet as they hit the ground, for example, or on your abdomen as it moves with your breath.

Visualization
Visualization, or imagining through any of the senses, can be used to make the run easier, to make you feel lighter and quicker, and to aid you in reaching a more playful or meditative state. You can try the following ones, or make up your own.

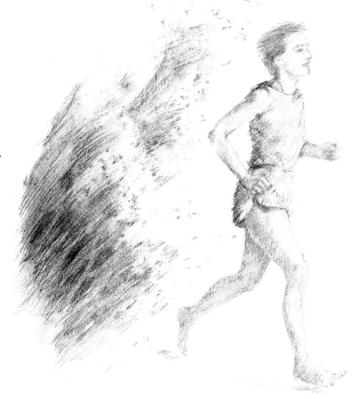

To create effortlessness, lightness, and ease, imagine being gently carried forward by a large wave at your back. Allow it to push you, lift you, carry you, and keep you clean, cool, and fresh.

Imagine yourself as a still, small point, moving quietly and effortlessly forward through space.

Feel your legs as perpetual motion pistons made of strongest iron, tirelessly carrying you forward.

Cooling down

It is vital to take the time to cool down after your run, to slow your body down and observe the internal experience of your run. Use the time while you stretch to pay attention to your feelings and sensations. Notice your muscles, your skin, and breathing, your pounding heart, and increased temperature. Notice any aches or soreness. Be aware of your attitudes, feelings, and thoughts. Once again, be patient with yourself and give yourself time. Remember to keep breathing, to release your weight into gravity, and to relax as many muscles as possible.

After your run...
Walk for 5 to 10 minutes.
Shake out your shoulders, hands, and feet.
Do 1 repetition each of the following warm-up exercises (see pp. 140-1):
Calf and hamstring stretch
Thigh stretch
Dorsal stretch
Now do the exercises below.

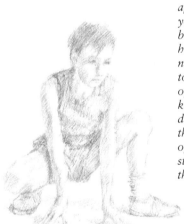

Hip stretch
(1 min, 5-15 reps)
Stand with feet hip-width apart. Squat down and place your hands on the floor between your feet, letting your heels lift off the floor if necessary. Gently rock 1 knee toward the floor, while opening and pressing the other knee backward. Alternately drop 1 knee to the ground and then the other, pressing the opposite knee back to create a stretch in the groin and inner thigh.

Runner's stretch
(2 mins, once each side)
With 1 knee bent and 1 leg outstretched behind you, turn so that you are facing over your bent leg, back leg extended, knee straight, heel pressing toward the wall behind you. Use your hands to support your weight. Allow gravity to pull your pelvis and hips down to the floor as you relax into the stretch. Repeat on the other side.

Relaxation
(3 mins)
Sit quietly and focus on your breath. Notice how you feel.

PARTNERWORK

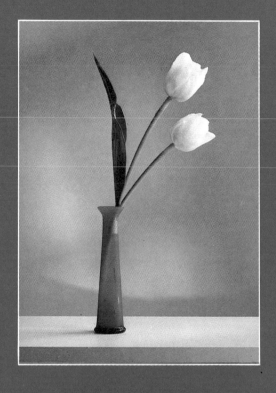

Harmonizing energies
Aikido

Taking up a form of bodywork that involves working with a partner can teach you a lot about the way you relate to others, and provide invaluable feedback in the process of self-development. The Japanese martial art Aikido is an ideal method of learning how to retain your own sense of inner balance and centeredness when with others, and how to harmonize your energy with your partner's. Founded by Morihei Ueshiba (1883-1969), it derives from the ancient fighting arts, which prized among their warriors cultivation of a dauntless spirit, oneness of intuition and action, and a need for awareness at every moment. In Aikido, Ueshiba sought to provide a practical and creative source of inspiration for cultivating peace and harmony, while retaining the spirit of the old fighting arts. The word itself is made up of three Japanese characters: *ai* (harmony), *ki* (the vital life force, also known as *chi*) and *do* (way). Thus one can translate Aikido as the way of harmony with *ki*, or the way of spiritual harmony.

In practising Aikido, the aim is not to beat, overpower, or dominate your partner, but instead to achieve total co-ordination of mind, body, and *ki*. Working with a partner, the techniques of Aikido allow you to explore and overcome any tendency to be either excessively dominating or too yielding. For Aikido is a concrete manifestation of the principle of *yin* and *yang*, or complementary opposites. It teaches you to be both "rock" and "water" – the rock around which the water must flow, and the water which seeks the way of least resistance. The concepts of conflict and struggle, of winning and losing, give way to a resolution of a higher order, both on a personal level and in relationships with others. Through training of mind and body, you move toward harmonizing the individual *ki* with the universal *ki*, a task shared with your partner. This unity finds expression in the flowing, spontaneous and powerful movements that are Aikido's hallmark.

As a beginner to the art, its apparently limitless range of techniques and subtle body movements can be baffling. However, after even a short period of practice, the basic principles of a centered, circular movement that absorbs, merges with, and leads the energy of your partner, reveal themselves. As your body becomes more centered and supple, you achieve in turn a growing self-confidence and a calm centeredness of mind, making you capable of clear, powerful, and creative involvement with the world in which you live.

In this chapter we present exercises which contain the fundamental principles of Aikido. These exercises are taught on the first day you become a student, and are refined at every practice. Infinitely subtle, yet infinitely revealing, it is said that if you master them, you master the art of Aikido.

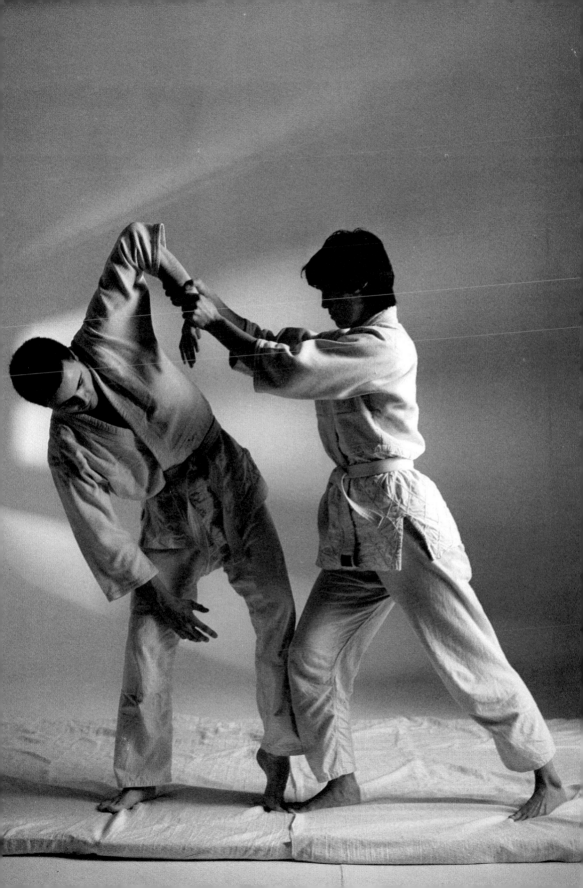

Kokyu – *unity with the ground*

Central to Aikido is the concept of *kokyu*. *Kokyu* can be defined as "breath power"; it can also describe the quality of the movement of your *ki*. To have "strong *kokyu*" denotes a profound connection to, and understanding of, the nature of the universe and your place in it. The first consideration when learning to develop *kokyu* is to perfect your stance or posture, which reveals the degree of your connection to the ground. With a strong, stable stance you take power and energy from the ground into your body, and extend "full *ki*" into everything you do. Many uncertainties and fears arise from lack of a strong, connecting stance: you are easily thrown "off centre", taken by surprise, distracted, and disoriented. A firm, balanced stance allows you to respond instantly to, and harmonize with, changes in the environment, both on a physical and mental plane.

"The essence of Aikido is the mutual echoing of the body with the resonance of the universe."
Morihei Ueshiba

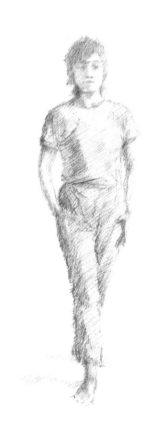

Kamae – *the posture*
The correct posture, known as kamae, *ensures maximum stability and projection of strong* ki, *and allows rapid movement in any direction.*

Stand with your right foot forward, front leg bent, back leg straight and braced into the ground, feet at right angles to each other. Angle your right hip and shoulder forward.

Now breathe into the abdomen, shoulders relaxed. Keep your arms by your sides, hands open, fingers filled with ki. *Repeat with the left foot forward.*

This strong, angled posture induces the correct mental attitude of preparedness and stability.

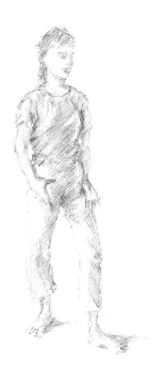

This exercise allows you to experience a profound connection to the ground, while at the same time extending your ki or energy outward. Let go of any tension in your arms and shoulders, as this will inhibit the stream of ki. You will need a partner to complete the exercise.

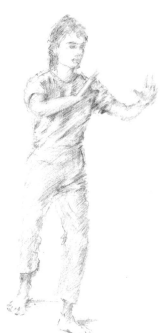

Assume kamae (see opposite). Breathe in, then exhale as you raise your arms, keeping them aligned with your hips. Move your front foot slightly forward as the knee and hip angle more deeply. Keep your fingers open, blades or outside edges of the hands turned slightly out. Finish with your arms at shoulder height.

With practice, you will feel an unbroken stream of energy travelling through your legs into the ground and coming up from the ground to pour out through the blades of your hands. Let your partner grasp your wrist and push toward your centre, into the ground. You should feel solid, and without tension.

Repeat the exercise, switching to the other foot forward.

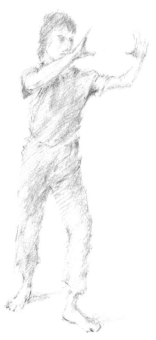

Kokyu – *breath power*

"Breath power" originates in the lower abdomen or centre – known as the *hara* in Japanese or *tan'tien* in Chinese. The *hara* is said to be the intersection of mind and body, allowing them to act as one. In all Aikido exercises you breathe in fully, then breathe out as you extend *ki* and execute the move. In using breath power, you begin to find your body working in a more co-ordinated fashion, and in unison with your intentions. As you breathe out, you learn to flow like water around your partner's energy, merging rather than colliding with it. In emphasizing power that originates in a strong centre or *hara*, breath power is in sharp contrast to muscular power, from the shoulders and arms. When power comes from the upper body, your centre of gravity is high, and you are more easily "thrown". Breath power indicates a state of alert relaxedness, a low and stable centre of gravity, and the ability to flow with the energy around you, while maintaining a strong centre. It opens the way to tremendous reserves of power, and the potential for creative action and fullness of being.

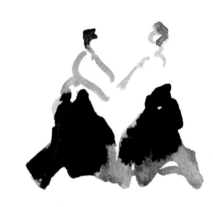

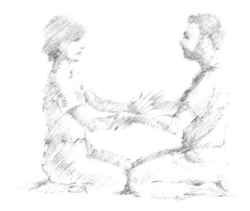

Kneel facing your partner, knee to knee (as shown right), your legs forming a triangular base, big toes crossing at the back.

Now raise your arms to chest height, hands held palms inward, about shoulder-width apart. Keep your shoulders and arms relaxed and your fingers open, so that power from the ground and centre can flow through your fingertips and beyond.

Let your partner grasp you lightly from the side, just above the wrists. Notice the curve of the arm. This is known as the

"unbendable arm", and serves as a direct channel for power coming from the centre, or hara.

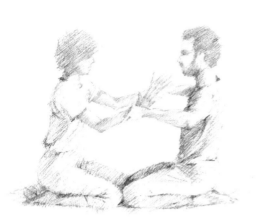

From this position use breath power to flow around your partner's strength. If you push straight in, for example, you will collide with that strength. If you pull, you will be easily restricted. Simply breathe in, turning the palms of your hands slightly upward and outward, then, keeping contact with the ground, breathe out and push your pelvis forward. Your arms will channel that movement to your partner.

As you push forward, your fingers turn up and your palms turn toward your partner's chest. Allow the blade of your hand to follow the natural curve of your partner's arm upward into the shoulder. Your partner should not let his or her grip adjust or slip. If your arms keep their "unbendable" form, you will maintain contact with your centre and the ground. Your partner's balance will now be taken back.

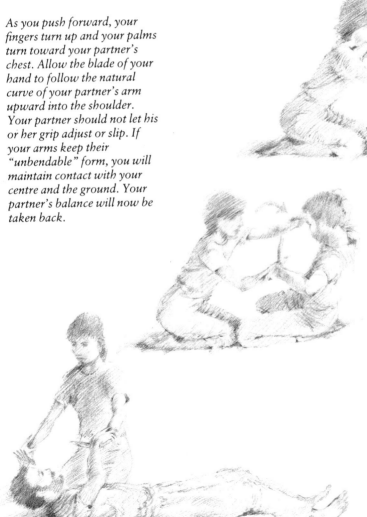

From here it is easy to guide your partner by pushing gently to the right (or left), allowing him or her to fall. As your partner falls, your toes come up and you follow, left (or right) knee into his or her armpit.

Now sit on your heels, toes up, with your centre over your partner, controlling his or her natural inclination to sit up. Practise this the other way around also, so you can experience being both the active and the yielding partner.

Kokyu – *non-resistance*

Non-resistance is a key feature of *kokyu*. Force meeting force, ego against ego, creates conflict and struggle. A competitive, aggressive spirit draws the same from those around it; so, by contrast, does a shrinking spirit that yields its own integrity or centre, attracting aggressive energy from its surroundings. Aikido techniques are not based on strength or brute force, but on an understanding of the structure of the human body and the laws that govern energy in all its manifestations. Situations of potential conflict are diverted into non-destructive, creative resolution. Even in these apparently simple exercises, you will find that an inclination to struggle to achieve the pictured movement will emerge. Work with that feeling without judgement. With sincere practice, you will become less distracted by your partner's energy. For in Aikido, you do not struggle against force, but seek out what is free from restriction and use that. Relax into your own centre, and use breath power to flow around rather than collide with your partner.

3. Take your right foot back so that you are shoulder to shoulder, arms extended easily from the hip, palms up and fingers open. You are in kamae, *front knee bent, back leg straight, braced into the ground. If your partner pulls back into your centre, you remain as solid as the ground beneath you. Repeat several times, reversing your positions.*

Tai no henko – *turning exercise*
1. Begin in kamae, *left foot and hand forward. Let your partner, also in* kamae, *grasp you firmly just above the wrist with his or her right hand.*

2. First, bend the wrist, aligning your hand with your partner's arm and its line of power. Pivoting on the balls of your feet, turn your hips to face in the same direction as your partner, blending with the direction of his or her energy.

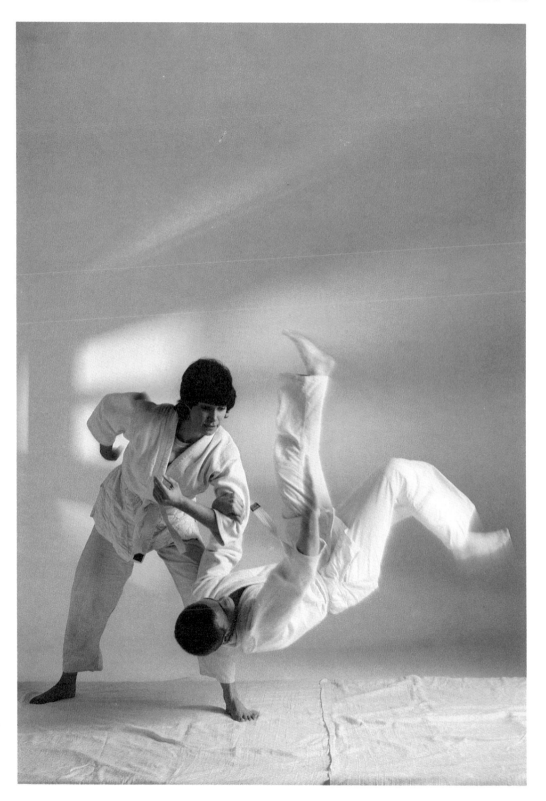

Kokyu – *harmonizing*

In choral song, voices join together in harmony to create something quite different to a voice on its own. To achieve fluid movement with your partner, you strive to become totally aware, and base your actions on the principles of harmony. In Aikido, to move your partner, you seek to discover the easiest angle that will not collide with the direction of your partner's strength and energy but, rather, merge and harmonize with them. At the same time you must strive to develop the integrity of your own "voice" – your own internal harmony that unites the powers of body and mind, unblocking internal tension or confusion.

Aikido is based on sound physical principles – principles that govern and animate all things in nature. Ueshiba once spoke of the movements of Aikido as the "materialization in minute detail of the movement of Heaven, Earth, and other aspects of Great Nature". Aikido can become a mirror for you – as you come to know it, you come to know yourself and others. The clearer the mirror, the more in harmony you are with your own fundamental nature and the nature of the world about you.

2. Bring your right hand up under the underarm, pushing your partner's elbow over his or her head. Your partner yields.

Ikkyo undo
In ikkyo undo, *you use your body movement to explore losing and regaining balance, in harmony with your partner.*

1. Begin with both of you in kamae, *left foot and hand forward. Advance your left foot, pushing your hand toward your partner's face.*

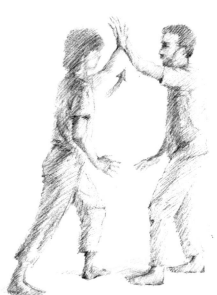

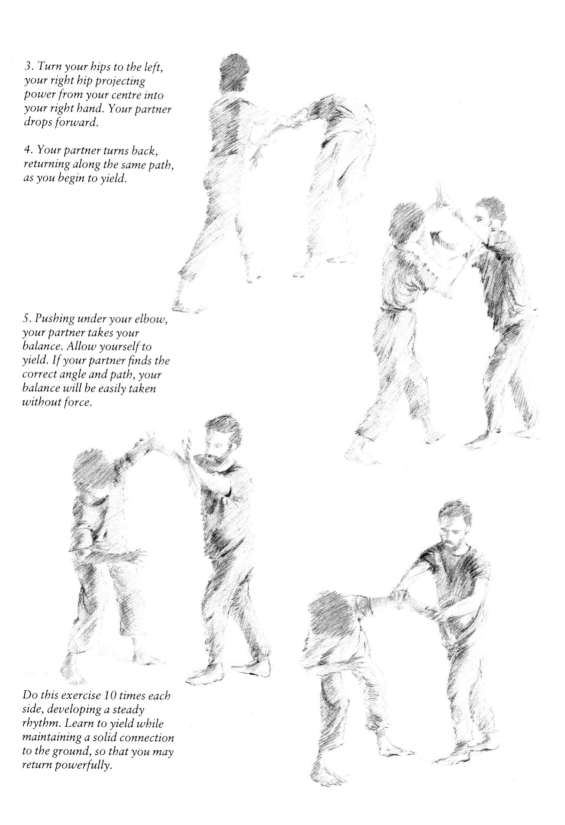

3. *Turn your hips to the left, your right hip projecting power from your centre into your right hand. Your partner drops forward.*

4. *Your partner turns back, returning along the same path, as you begin to yield.*

5. *Pushing under your elbow, your partner takes your balance. Allow yourself to yield. If your partner finds the correct angle and path, your balance will be easily taken without force.*

Do this exercise 10 times each side, developing a steady rhythm. Learn to yield while maintaining a solid connection to the ground, so that you may return powerfully.

Kokyu – *mind and body as one*

With continued practice in Aikido, as your mind and
body begin to work as one unit, you come to
experience yourself as a whole person and to find a
natural way of being in the world that is expressive,
positive, and without struggle or uncertainty. You
begin, for example, to make decisions not just with
your mind, but with your whole being – body and
mind moving together from the centre. Conflicts are
often created by the need to win, to demonstrate
superior power and ability to exert brute force.
Without the need to win, or the fear of losing, you
begin to engage creatively with what is – physically,
mentally, and spiritually.

Learning to breakfall allows you to practise some
of the more powerful Aikido techniques. It pushes
back your own limits, opening you up to a broader
spectrum of experience. You begin to unlock your
own power, learning to develop and use it freely and
creatively. In the breakfall, you discover how to relax
and trust the ground to break your fall without fear.
Your body becomes soft, resilient, and strengthened
by your ability to fall and spring up from the ground.

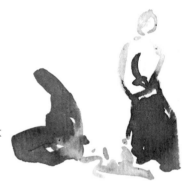

Ukemi – *the breakfall*
*On a soft surface, step back on
your left foot, as shown above.
Lower your body on to your
left heel, holding your arms in
front of you. Curve your back
and tuck your chin in.*

*Now roll backward, keeping
yourself tucked into a ball,
arms held in front for balance
and to avoid hitting your
elbows on the ground.*

*Allow the momentum of the
roll to take you back and then
rock you forward.
Stand up, without using your
hands to push yourself up.
Resume a balanced posture.*

Sumi otoshi – *a throw*
Assume kamae, *right foot and hand forward. Your partner, with left side forward, grasps your arm just above your wrist with his or her left hand.*

Dropping your hip and bending your right knee, lower your centre, taking the palm of your hand toward the ground. Keep your arm in contact with your centre. There should be no feeling of tugging your partner.

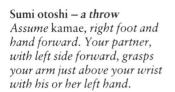

With your right foot, take a sliding step to your partner's rear, allowing your back foot to follow. To the rear your partner has no support, and will not be able to resist the throw.

Your partner breakfalls on the foot furthest from you, as the near foot could be trapped.

Relating

It is in close relationships that our whole way of being is revealed most clearly and tested most critically. Relating to our partners calls into question the most fundamental issues: how can you avoid losing your sense of self when with another? Can you divide your attention between your own needs and those of your partner, between giving and taking? How can you keep the lines of communication open? Can you maintain a balance where neither of you needs to take or surrender too much personal space and power?

How well or poorly we relate to others depends largely on the kinds of experiences we had while growing up. If we had parents who loved and accepted us, who understood what we needed and trusted us to make our own choices, then we are more likely to grow up into confident, creative, emotionally well-balanced adults, for whom relating to others seems a challenge. But if in childhood our needs were poorly understood and we were discouraged from expressing our feelings or choosing for ourselves, then problems may recur in close relationships later on in life. Since few people had a *perfect* childhood, most of us need to be prepared to learn how to improve the way we relate in adult life.

Honesty is essential if our relationships are to be lasting and mutually fulfilling – many couples become distanced from one another by withholding their true feelings. Some people also have problems in sharing their feelings because they themselves no longer know how they feel, having spent so many years pretending to be different from how they really are.

Surprisingly, perhaps, one of the best ways of making our relationships more fulfilling is by working on ourselves – learning to trust and enjoy our own bodies, to be more in touch with ourselves. If you have a good sense of yourself and are at home in your body, in contact with your feelings, and aware of your own needs, you are far more likely to make a good relationship than if you are constantly looking for your partner to give you confidence, approval, or reassurance. The best relationships are those in which both partners feel secure and able to trust themselves, as well as one another.

The exercises in this chapter will show you both how much trust and openness there is in your relationship, and help you to extend your trust and understanding of one another through communicating more clearly. Some of the exercises derive from co-counselling, a practical method of personal development designed to help you to become aware of and release painful feelings and increase your enjoyment in life. But since successful relationships are so much a matter of how well you relate to yourself, you will also find useful advice in the Solowork section of the book.

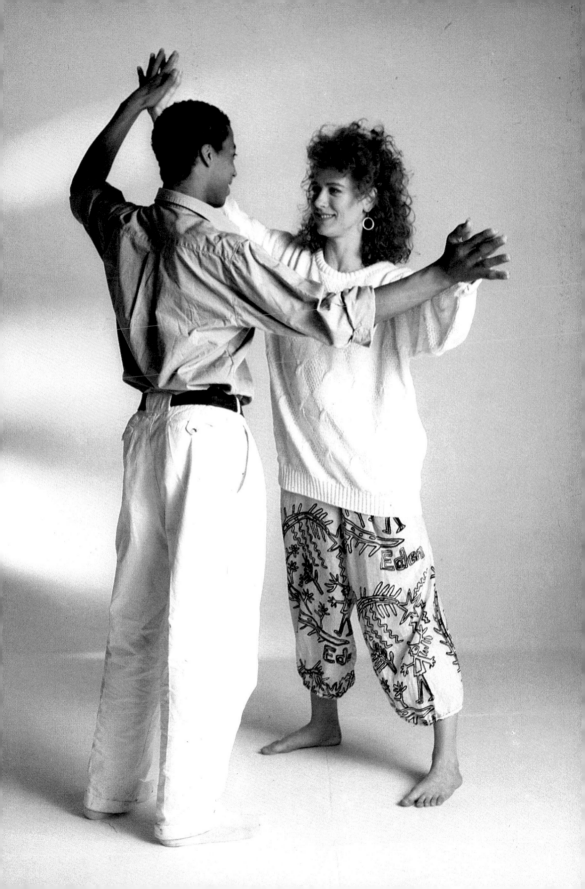

Vulnerability and trust

As children, all too many of us learn to armour
ourselves against the world, to develop a tough outer
shell, as a way of surviving and protecting our
vulnerability. In adult life, we endeavour to keep the
armour in place by controlling our emotions, refusing
to share feelings of vulnerability, or withholding our
trust. Nowhere is this more damaging than in an
intimate relationship. If you are to develop any degree
of closeness and trust between you, it's essential to
recognize your armouring and begin to open
yourselves up to one another. Paradoxically, learning
to lay down the armour that we use to protect
ourselves and allowing ourselves to share feelings of
hurt or loss or anger, lead to the development of a
new kind of strength, deepening and enriching your
relationship. By daring to be vulnerable and to free
yourself from rigid self-control, you will also free the
flow of love between you. The following exercises
make use of body language to discover how ready
you are to share your vulnerability. They can show
you more about how you relate to one another than
any amount of verbal discussion.

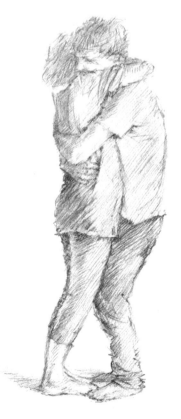

Hugging
*The way you hug each other
can tell you a lot about the way
you relate – how much you are
willing to relinquish control
and give yourself to one
another, how open you are to
letting your partner in. Do you
melt into each other? Are
either of you rigid or unyield-
ing? Do you crush your partner or feel crushed? Are either
of you avoiding genital contact? Next time you embrace
your partner, see if you can
improve the way you hug.*

*Try moving slowly toward
your partner and putting your
arms around him or her. Try,
also, running toward your
partner and flinging your arms
around him or her. Make as
much body contact as you can,
remembering that the essence
of good hugging is to hold
close without grasping.*

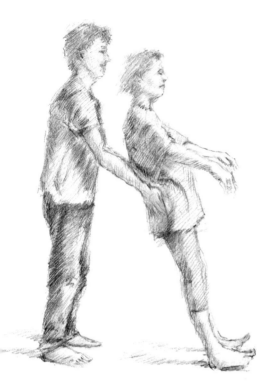

Falling and catching

Falling blindly into someone else's arms involves a very basic kind of trust. You may at first find it difficult to let go of that much control. Take your time to do the exercise, and only fall when you feel ready. Stand about 2 feet in front of your partner. Close your eyes and, in your own time, let yourself fall backward to be caught by him or her. Now swap roles. If you can let yourself fall quite easily, make it a little more challenging by counting to 30 with your eyes closed, before falling.

Rag doll

Since many of us associate being vulnerable with losing control of ourselves and our emotions, we may hold ourselves back too much and find it difficult to let go of the reins when the need for control is removed. In this exercise you go to the opposite extreme of overcontrol, allowing yourself to become completely floppy, like a rag doll.

Sit down on the floor, with your partner kneeling behind you, and lean back against him or her. Allow yourself to go completely limp, and let your partner lift your hands and arms and move them freely in any direction they will go. With a minimum of co-operation, let your partner lift you slowly and carefully to your feet and walk you about the room, moving your arms and legs as necessary. After a while, swap roles. Were you equally comfortable in either role or did you find it easier being the active or passive partner?

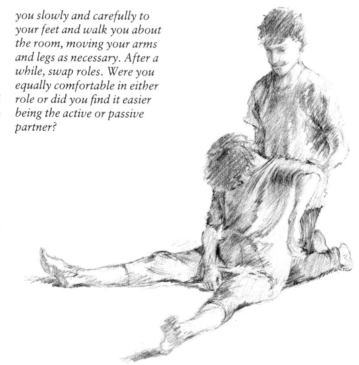

Active listening and looking

Giving our full, undivided attention to someone is one of the greatest gifts we can bestow. All too often, conversation takes the form of a contest, a verbal tennis match in which we compete with each other to score points by the speed and wit of our responses, or use the time when the other person is talking to work out a reply. Active or "open" listening means developing a more alert way of giving your full attention to what someone is saying. As the listener you simply sit back and listen, alert and interested, but without responding in any way to what the speaker is saying. This gives the speaker the space to be open and creative, to explore what he or she feels or thinks, without needing to compete for attention, and without being interrupted or feeling judged by the listener. The first few times you try it, adopt a slightly formal approach. Sit facing one another and agree how much time you have, who will talk first, and whether what is said is to be confidential between you. Then just listen while your partner talks about his or her problems, discoveries, anxieties, and so on. Be sure to take the same amount of time when it's your turn to speak.

Maintaining eye contact

We undoubtedly feel the strongest connection with people when we look directly into their eyes. But frequently we avoid or limit eye contact, repeatedly averting our gaze while we speak. For the eyes reveal our true feelings and maintaining eye contact means coming out of hiding, laying our inner state open to another. Learning to prolong eye contact involves daring to be more honest, being willing to allow another person in. It also brings us into the present moment, and shows us how much attention we are actually able to give. Try holding eye contact with your partner while you talk, maintaining a light, steady gaze, not an unblinking stare. Experiment, too, with gazing at one another for a few minutes without talking.

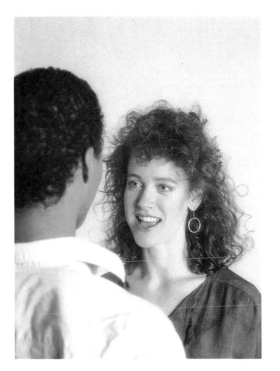
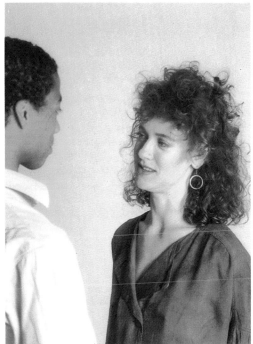
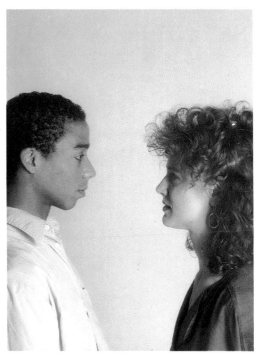
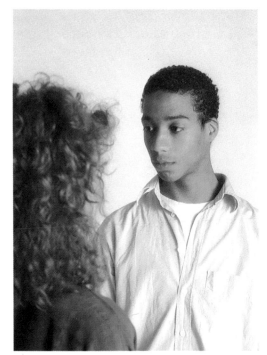

Clear communication

In order to develop deep, lasting relationships, it's essential to learn to understand and express yourself clearly. Knowing how to communicate strong negative or positive feelings without hostility or embarrassment, to say both "yes" and "no" and mean it, are vital for relating well to your partner. In many relationships, however, communicating negative feelings is often avoided altogether, or else you may find yourselves either "pussy footing", saying less than you intend, or "sledge-hammering", being damagingly critical. The only way we are likely to be heard by our partners is if we air our objections or complaints from a loving position, using a genuinely affectionate tone. One way of doing this is to match each of your negative statements with an appreciative remark. Next time you feel resentful or critical of your partner, sit down together and first say what you appreciate about him or her. Then, taking equal time, talk about the ways in which you feel hurt or neglected or what you resent about his or her behaviour. As in active listening (p.162), there should be no response from your partner while you are talking.

I see, I imagine, I feel

Taking responsibility for what we feel rather than blaming our partners is another important feature of relating in a clear, adult way. It's vital to be able to distinguish between what we *perceive* our partners to be doing, what we *imagine* to be going on, and what we *feel* about it. If you *see* your partner throwing something down on the floor, for example, you may *imagine* that he or she is angry and *feel* worried that you are going to be criticized – when, in fact, neither your fantasy nor your feeling may correspond to the reality of the situation. Any time a disagreement looks like escalating between you, try to slow down and apply this formula. By recognizing that your perceptions, ideas, or feelings may not represent the whole truth, you can learn how large a part fantasy plays in relationships, and avoid misunderstandings.

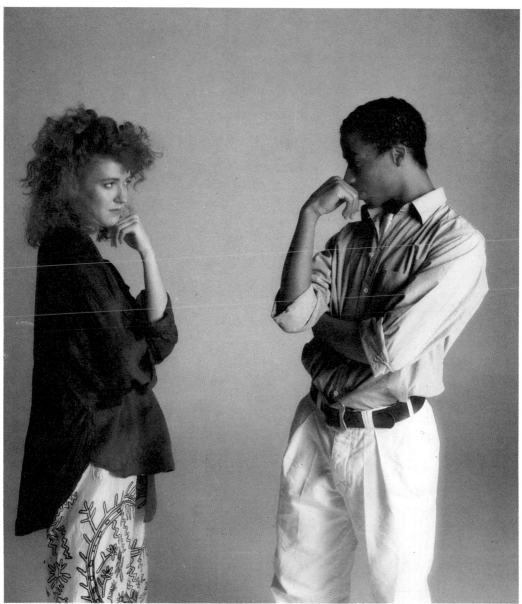

Mirroring

Your body tends to reveal your feelings, even though you may deny them verbally. For example, you may insist that "no, you are not angry", while your body expresses the opposite. Mirroring is a way of discovering what your gestures, posture, and mannerisms reveal about you. While you talk to your partner, ask him or her to mirror your body language, precisely as it happens, without judgement or exaggeration. This may make you acutely self-conscious at first, because you are being made aware of behaviour of which you were previously unconscious. But if you persevere with it, you can learn a lot from your partner's feedback about the messages you are unconsciously transmitting through your body language. After a while, swap roles.

Releasing trapped energy

In childhood, situations often occur which seem to throw into doubt our whole survival as a person – painful situations such as going into hospital, bullying, or the loss of one of our parents. What we did at that time to survive such threats to us as a person – fighting back, giving up, or withdrawing – is likely to be trapped as an imprint in our bodymind. This part of our personal history, frozen in our bodies, lies there ready to be triggered if some trauma arises in the present that resembles the earlier situation. Faced with a stern, domineering person, for example, who unconsciously reminds us of a teacher we feared at school, we may become inexplicably indecisive. But while bringing childhood memories and feelings to the surface can be disturbing, simply to make the connection between our behaviour in the present and the survival decision that started it off is often very rewarding.

In a relationship, such unresolved experiences from your childhood can come between you and your partner, causing you to be unduly aggressive at times, perhaps, or to appear unintentionally cold or cut off. In addition, you may go through periods of feeling alienated from one another if one of you finds it difficult to get in touch with his or her feelings. On such occasions it's good to have a way of discharging your feelings of anger or frustration, rather than venting them on your partner, who may have done nothing to cause them. On the following pages we look at various techniques that can help you to release the energy trapped in your body and let go of your feelings. In doing any of the exercises, if you feel yourself becoming overwhelmed by feelings that you can't handle, you will be able safely to come back to your normal state of consciousness if you stand up, open your eyes (if they are closed), and describe in detail what you see around you. Counting objects in the room, books on the shelf, or listing the names of your friends or work-mates also works very well. For any of the techniques shown on the facing page, your partner should be present.

Stamping

Lightly at first, then with increasing energy, move about the room stamping your feet harder and harder. Put your whole weight into your stamping, feeling the resistance of the floor beneath your feet. Make a sound to go with the stamping. If you find this difficult, try repeating "I will" or "I won't", to begin with. Stamping is useful whenever a situation occurs in which you need to get in touch with and express feelings of anger and rage.

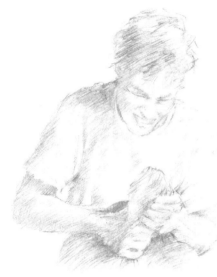

Wringing cushions

A good way of releasing your aggression is to wring a cushion or a rolled-up towel in both hands, putting all your strength into twisting it. Let yourself make any sound that feels right or repeat a phrase such as "I hate you" or "give it to me".

Temper tantrum

Lie on your back on a mattress, or on the floor with thick cushions under your hands and feet. Bend your knees. Now let a rising shout of "no, no" take you into repeatedly kicking and pounding with your hands and feet.

Caution Always do this when your partner is present, as it can put you in touch with strong feelings and evoke early memories. Your partner can help to bring you back to the present by suggesting one of the methods described opposite.

Talking nonsense and pulling faces

We often use words to rationalize away painful feelings or keep our "frozen history" quiet. To begin to bring negative feelings to the surface so we can get free of them, it's good to stop using words, transferring communication wholly to the body. Have a conversation in which you communicate only by jabbering and pulling faces. Try to keep it going past the point where you first want to stop, carrying on for at least 5 minutes. Give yourself permission to explore the extremes – from vigorous to gentle, loud to quiet. If you simply can't let yourself produce nonsense, make animal noises instead.

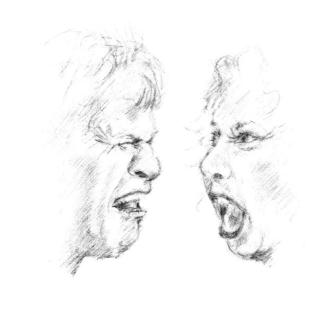

Yes/no – pushing across the floor

Releasing anger or resentment at not having been able to make our own choices and decisions in the past can be very rewarding, leading to a new vigour and capacity for zestful pleasure in the here and now. Sit back to back on the floor with your partner, preferably barefoot. Now try to push each other across to the opposite wall of the room. Shout with each push either "no" or "yes". By shouting "yes" or "no" at another person, you are learning to assert yourself. The exercise allows for the full expression of vigorous feelings, both positive and negative, so don't be surprised if it leads to an emotional release of some kind if you really throw yourself into it.

Caution These exercises are powerful. If you feel they are risky or might uncover too much too fast, it's best to leave them alone.

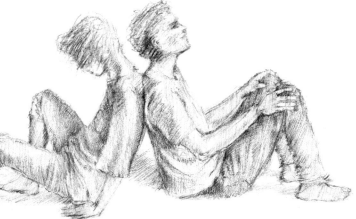

Other lives

For several hundred years, the way we relate to others has been immensely affected by the emphasis in our culture on manipulating, categorizing, and controlling people and things. In this view of reality the world is composed of separate, isolated objects and human beings. Today, however, this idea of reality is rapidly being replaced by another, more accurate one, which emphasizes the relationships between people and between things. This view shows that everything is connected to everything else, and that there is a global, planet-wide, social and political dimension to relating. We may ignore it, but we are connected anyway. Willingly or unwillingly, we move along on the tide of history. Seeing ourselves as part of a long thread of life, stretching back for millions of years, can lead to us treating ourselves and those around us with more tenderness and love. Devised by Joanna Macy, the following exercise (given here in a shortened version) is an effective way of beginning to experience the interconnections between the outer global and the inner personal aspects of ourselves, and of integrating our thinking capacity with what we feel.

Holding
For this "guided meditation", one partner lies down, while the other kneels by him or her. If you can, read the words on to a cassette recorder for playing back to both of you as you take turns.
"Take up your partner's left hand... feel the warmth in it... feel the strength in the fingers... this hand embodies millions of years of evolution. Now move on to your partner's left leg... lift it... feel the weight of the bone and muscle... this leg knows how to carry the body... think of the places that this foot has taken the person to whom it belongs. Now move on to the right leg... think of the life it has yet to support.

"Move to the right hand and arm...this hand has many skills... perhaps it plays music... delivers babies... prepares food.

"Now move to your partner's head... the brain inside this skull has within it a vast realm of experience... it may know several languages... write novels... treat this head tenderly... lay it down now gently, as you would a newborn child and, if you wish... bless it with a kiss."

Touching and pleasure
Sensual massage

Touch is the first of our senses to come into being. As infants, the loving touch of our parents reassures us that we are accepted and helps us to grow up with a feeling of our own self-worth. In early childhood we reach out instinctively toward pleasure – for love, comfort, and affection. If our needs are answered, our capacity for pleasure can survive and expand, but if our demands are met with frustration then our security is threatened, and pleasure becomes linked with pain. As a result we may withdraw and erect defences, diminishing feeling in parts of the body to reduce the anxiety and hurt.

As a couple you can help each other gradually to reclaim your natural capacity for pleasure through the use of sensual, loving touch. In all too many sexual relationships, touching and caressing play only a minimal role. But this is a real waste of our sensual potential. For the whole body can be erotic, and each of us has an individual body-map of pleasure to be explored together. Learning to enjoy and extend times of touching one another will also greatly enrich and intensify your lovemaking, for prolonged fondling and caressing stimulate the body's hormones, heightening arousal, so that when you do climax the energetic charge is far higher.

Leading into the sensual massage, we suggest two exercises aimed at deepening the feelings of intimacy and trust between you. You don't need any formal skills to give a sensual massage – it is simply an elaboration of what you might do normally as a prelude to making love. It differs from foreplay, however, in several important ways. Firstly, it involves one of you, the "receiver", being completely passive, while the other, the "giver", is active. Secondly, for the first few sessions, we recommend you make an agreement that the massage will not lead on to lovemaking. This frees the receiver to relax into enjoying the sensations of touch, without being distracted by thinking about performance or goals or the need to satisfy or be satisfied.

Many people find the experience of being caressed for an extended period even more intimate than lovemaking, and need to accustom themselves gradually to new dimensions of pleasure. When it is your turn to be receptive, try to keep your breathing constant – if you hold your breath you dampen your feelings of arousal. And focus your awareness entirely on the place that is being touched.

Before giving a sensual massage, take time to set the scene. Soften the lighting or use candles to create a relaxed atmosphere, and make sure your room is warm enough for you both to enjoy being naked. Using an oil or massage cream scented with some essential oil will help you to move more smoothly over your partner's body.

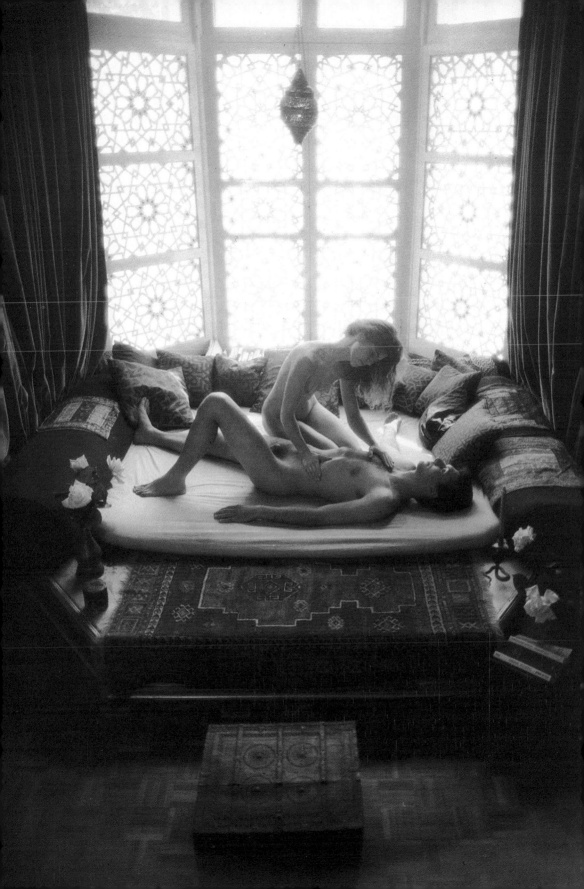

Gazing at one another

As children we are not afraid to stare at people, but as we grow up there is less and less opportunity to look at each other with such candour and curiosity. In adult life, the idea of being deliberately observed by another person tends to arouse feelings of acute shyness and self-consciousness, especially when we are naked. But in a close relationship, if you are to accept yourself and one another fully, it's essential not to keep parts of yourself hidden. Although you may see each other naked every day, purposely spending 15-30 minutes looking at one another can be a surprisingly intimate experience. In standing naked before the gaze of a loved one, you are daring to drop your mask and expose yourself completely, rather than hoping that those parts you may regard as "ugly" remain unseen by your partner. Allowing your eyes to linger as you carefully explore your partner's whole body, you learn to discover and appreciate one another exactly as you are, in all your uniqueness.

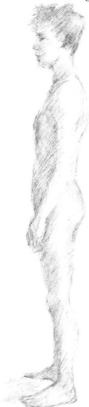

Take your clothes off and stand face to face, resting your hands on one another's shoulders. Close your eyes and begin to become aware first of your own then of your partner's breathing...

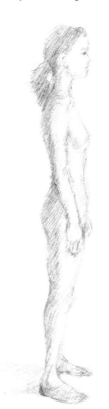

...After a few minutes, open your eyes, gently release your hands, and step back so you can observe your partner as a whole. Starting at the top of the head, begin to take in each other's body, gazing with curiosity at every detail...

...Observe the hair, then rest your gaze on the forehead, before making eye contact. Then slowly travel down the body, allowing yourself to really stare like a child at each part – face, neck, shoulders, arms, breasts, belly, genitals, and so on. Try, too, observing each other from the back and sides, in movement, or in different lighting.

Talking about your body

Even in an intimate relationship, we are often scared
to reveal feelings of inadequacy or self-doubt for fear
of alienating our partner. But it's important to be able
to open up fully, to trust yourself and your partner
enough to show your vulnerability – and in the long
run, sharing your true feelings will strengthen the
bond between you. In this exercise each of you in turn
talks about the parts of your body you like and
dislike, while the other listens. The "negative" parts
are generally those that cause pain or embarrassment
or those that we feel don't conform to a desired
stereotype. As the listener, your role is simply to give
your partner the space to talk about his or her
feelings, and, if necessary, to relive past hurts. Don't
be tempted to intervene and contradict what is said,
nor attempt to comfort your partner while he or she is
talking, as this can be suppressive and prevent a true
release of feelings. Wait until he or she has finished
before discussing anything that strikes you.
Surprisingly, it's often harder to talk about the parts
of yourself you appreciate, since many of us have
grown up with the ideal of modesty.

Talking about your body
Sit down facing one another.
Decide which of you will talk
first and which will listen. As
the speaker, begin by talking
about the parts of your body
you don't like, including any
fears or memories you
associate with them.

After hearing your partner's
feedback, talk about the parts
you like.

As the listener, wait until after
your partner has finished
speaking before sharing what
you observed or felt. When
you are ready, swap roles and
repeat the exercise.

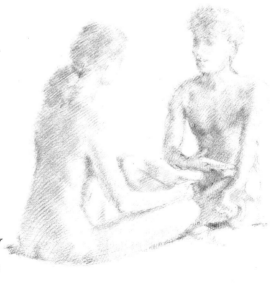

Sensual massage

In a close relationship, it is the quality of communication between you that counts above all else. Massage is a language without words, a two-way exchange of energy, demanding openness and receptivity on the part of both giver and receiver. As the giver your role is to awaken your partner, through the sensitivity of your touch, to his or her capacity for pleasure. In your eagerness to please your partner, however, don't overlook your own enjoyment, for it's impossible to touch sensitively if the pleasure is one-sided. Keep your breathing and posture relaxed, and move your hands slowly and gently, following the curves and forms of the body. Feel the different textures of the body and the warmth and electricity of the skin, and let the sensations of pleasure flow through you too. Closing your eyes will help you to sense with your hands what your partner's body likes best. When receiving massage too, for the first few sessions, you should keep your eyes closed. In time, however, you can learn to enjoy your partner's touch with open eyes, without being distracted from your own sensations.

Attuning
When you are ready to begin the massage, start by sitting down facing one another. Be aware of your contact with the floor. Relax your shoulders and face and simply feel your breath coming in and out.

When you feel relaxed, allow your hands to meet your partner's. Hold your left hand palm up and your right hand palm down and let your middle fingers rest on the centre of your partner's palms. Close your eyes and just sit there together for a while, feeling the energy flowing between your 2 beings.

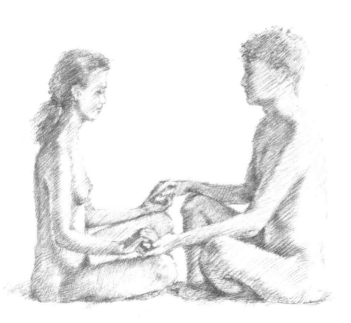

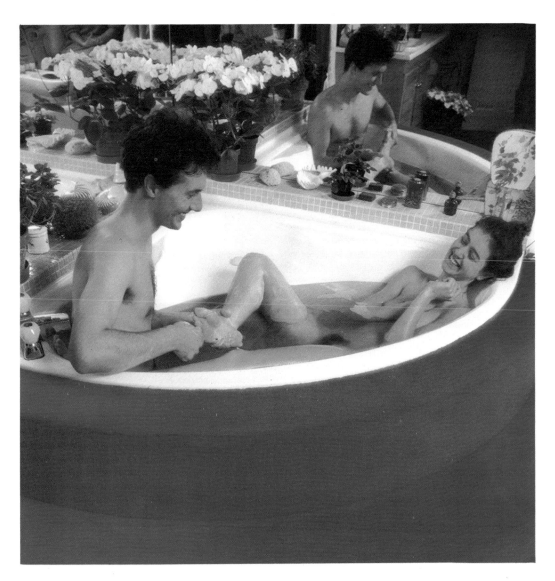

Sharing a bath
As a way of getting closer and more relaxed prior to a massage – or simply for the fun of it – there's no substitute for sharing a hot bath or shower with your partner. It's a rare pleasure to wash or be washed by someone else and you can use fragrant liquid soap or essential oils to heighten the sensuality of the whole experience.

Beginning a massage

For the receiver in a sensual massage, the accent is on
learning to let go and accept the intensity of
pleasurable sensations flowing through your body. As
the active partner, it's up to you to create a warm,
relaxing ambience. Soft music often enhances
relaxation and will also help you to glide your hands
rhythmically over your partner's body. Treat the
body with reverence, using whatever strokes feel right
for the part you are touching. Some people find light,
feathery, fingertip strokes most electric; for others,
firmer, broader strokes, made with the whole hand,
are more sensual. It's up to your partner to tell you
what feels good.

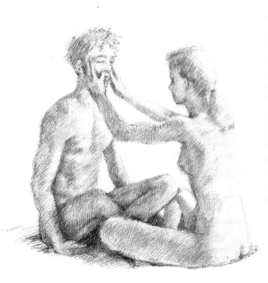

*Sitting opposite your partner,
gently explore his or her face
with your fingertips – across
the cheeks, around the eyes
and nose, over the lips, and
inside and behind the ears.
Touch very lightly, caressing
the whole face in the most
sensual and loving way you
can imagine. End by rapidly
rubbing your palms together to
build up heat, then placing
them over your partner's eyes
or ears.*

*Kneel down behind your
partner and gently massage the
scalp, neck, and shoulders.
Play with your partner's hair,
feeling its electricity and
texture, and slowly pull your
fingers off the ends. Stroke
gently down the back of the
head and neck and along the
shoulders, moulding your
hands to the contours of the
body.*

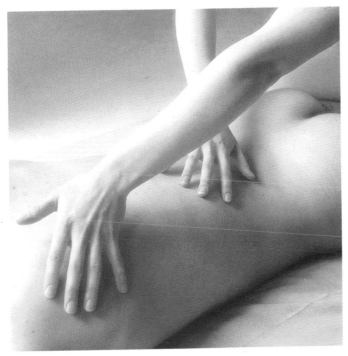

Straddling your partner's thighs is a perfect position from which to caress the whole of the back and buttocks. To oil the back, try moving both hands repeatedly up the spine then down the sides in a kind of breaststroke. Use your hands to make swirly patterns, as if trailing your fingers through sand or water. See how it feels to trace circles over the base of the spine with the flat of your hand, and try brushing your fingertips lightly down the whole of the back with one hand after the other.

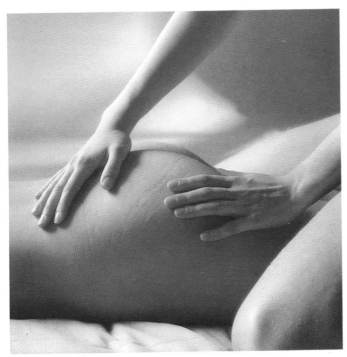

The buttocks are often one of the most responsive areas to touch. Some people enjoy a "kneading" stroke – using the "V" between thumbs and fingers to push with alternate hands up the buttocks from the tops of the thighs. Also, try shaking the buttocks from side to side and back and forth – with your hand pressed against the base of your partner's buttock crease. You might also like to stroke your fingertips repeatedly down the buttocks from the base of the back, with one hand after the other.

Kneeling between your partner's knees, use the whole of your hands to smooth oil into the backs of the legs, stroking softly up the inside of the legs from the ankles to the buttocks, then curving round the hip joints and drawing back down the outside of the legs and off the feet...

...The backs of the knees can be an unexpected source of delight.

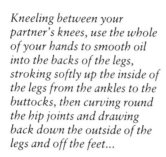

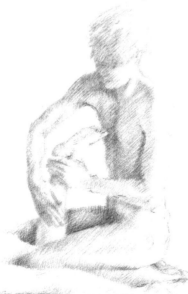

It feels very reassuring for the receiver if you enfold part of his or her body in your own. To stroke the lower leg, try bending the knee, lifting the foot, and kneeling down with your partner's knee firmly clasped between your knees. Rest the foot on your shoulder and glide your hands up and down the calf and shin, as if you were playing an instrument.

The ankles and soles of the feet can be highly erotic areas, very sensitive to the lightest touch. Sit or kneel down with your partner's foot across 1 of your thighs. Cradle the toes in 1

hand while you caress the sole and spiral round the sculpted shapes of the ankle and heel with your fingertips. Using plenty of oil, try also sliding a finger in and out between each

pair of toes. End by brushing down the sole from heel to toes, with light feathery strokes.

A good position for stroking
the front of the body is to sit
back against a pile of cushions,
with your partner enfolded
securely between your legs.
With your partner's back
resting against your chest,
stroke gently up the belly
and chest, and around or over
the breasts. Explore the
contours and textures with
your most sensual touch,
brushing over but not lingering
on the nipples.

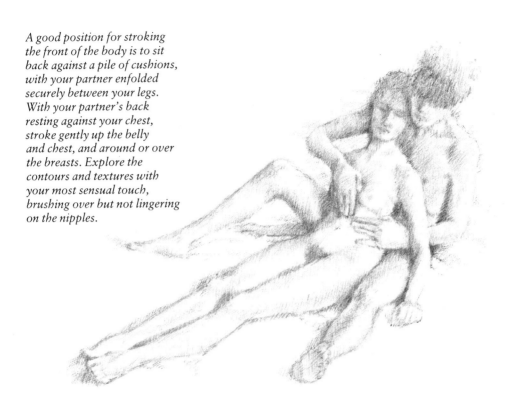

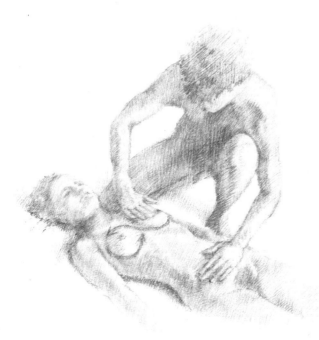

Kneel or sit down at your
partner's side and place one
hand over the hara, on the
lower belly. With the other
hand, trace a delicate figure of
eight shape around the breasts.
To give the greatest pleasure,
your touch should be soft and
soothing and the movement
repeated continuously for a
good few moments.

To caress the arms and hands,
sit or kneel by your partner's
side, facing the head. Glide
your oiled hands up the centre
of the arm from the wrist,
separating them briefly at the
top of the arm so that 1 travels
around the shoulder and the
other curves around the
armpit, exploring the
underarm hollow. Then enfold
the arm in both palms as you
draw back down its long
curves and off the hand. Trace
the outlines of the hand, and
stroke your partner's palm
softly with your fingertips,
then slowly slide your hands
off each finger in turn.

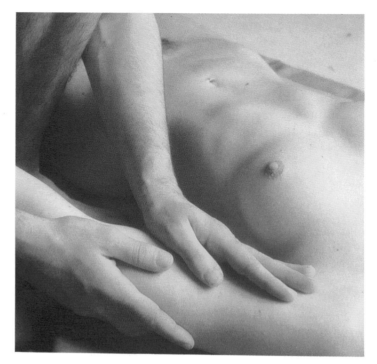

Let your hands come to rest
very gently on your partner's
belly and leave them there
without moving for a few
moments. Then slowly start to
draw light circles around the
belly, gliding over the contours
of flesh in a clockwise
direction, with 1 hand
following the other.

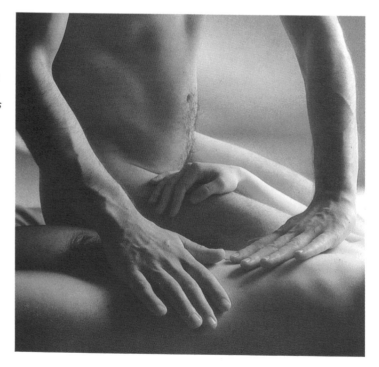

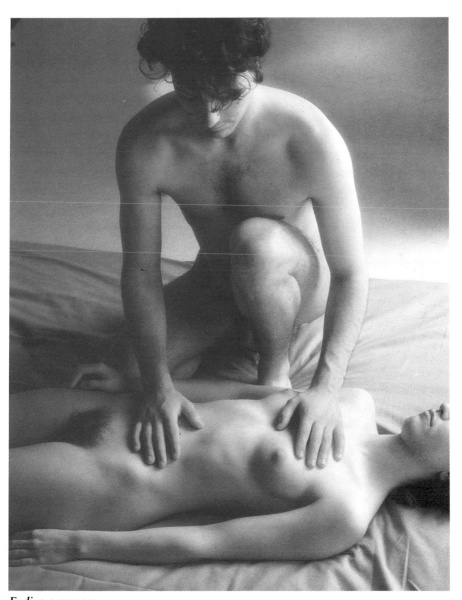

Ending a massage

When you have finished, you need to end with some long, connecting strokes, to leave your partner's body feeling whole. Using the fingertips, start by resting your hands on the belly, then glide 1 hand up the torso and down 1 arm and the other down 1 leg. Do this on both sides of the body. You can also connect by simply resting each hand on a different part of the body, such as chest and belly, or belly and forehead. After connecting, cover your partner with a rug or a warmed towel, allowing him or her to bask in the afterglow of pleasure.

The loving body

Nowhere is our disconnectedness from the body more distressingly evident than in our attitude to sex. Divorced from our instinctive nature, sex has become a matter of "performance" and "goals", relegated to the province of our minds. In addition, our cultural heritage has conditioned us to see only the mind as capable of divine perceptions and to regard our bodies and our sexual drives as an impediment to spiritual development. In tantric yoga, by contrast, the union of two people in sexual love is used as an instrument to increase self-awareness, as a path to divine union.

"Being more alive means being more sexual, more sensuous. To be more sexual is to broaden one's range of feeling and expressive action."
Stanley Keleman

Within our western culture, there are still many who are fearful of revealing the body's inherent sensuality. Uprooted from our basic biological and bodily ground, we have tended to deny our "animal" nature, downgrading it in relation to the mind. As a result, when we come to make love, we find it hard to give full rein to our instincts and our heads often take the leading role. Only when we begin to heal this split and to live more totally in our whole beings, uniting our instinctual, emotional, spiritual, and mental selves, will we be able fully to enjoy and express our sexuality.

In the act of love we can experience ourselves in our wholeness, body, heart, and soul united with another being. To allow the deeper feelings and pulsations of desire to flower in an organic way requires a willingness to drop our façades, to allow ourselves to be open and vulnerable. But in order to let go we need above all to be able to trust one another.

Learning how to experience more pleasure in your lovemaking will naturally evolve from sharing in sensual massage. But you also need to stay in the moment, not forcing the pace, to listen to your body, and to be able to communicate your feelings and individual preferences. Ultimately, it is only in an atmosphere of love, warmth, and mutual respect that sex becomes deeply fulfilling on all levels of our being.

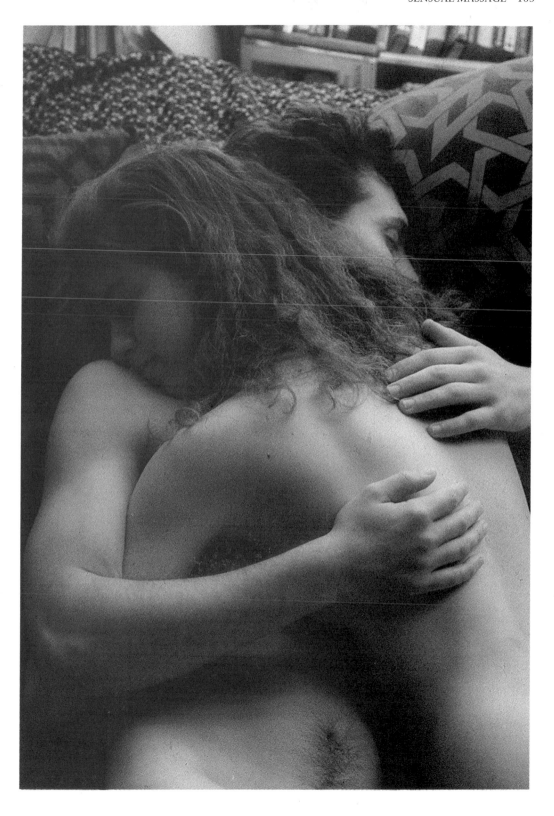

Awakening

The more in touch we become with ourselves, the more we can come in touch with the reality and experience of the world around us. Once we begin to inhabit our bodies, then we can begin truly to inhabit this planet in which we live.

If you are not aware of yourself as a whole, integrated being – a unity of body, mind, and spirit – it is difficult to perceive the unity of all nature. And the divided, fragmented self is mirrored in the divisions and increasing fragmentation of the global human community today. We forget that we are all members of one family, all creatures of one beginning, that we share our breath with all other living things, and the atoms in our bodies with the atoms of stars and galaxies.

Living in cities, it is easy to feel separate from nature, to lose contact with the earth under our feet, the sun and wind, the touch of rain. But few of us are aware of how much we lose by this. By becoming estranged from the natural world, we begin to lose contact with what we are, and to feel alienated from our own beings.

In becoming habitually desensitized and deadened to our physical experience, we cut ourselves off too from real feeling and compassion for the world around us – the degradation of our living planet, and the sufferings of other human beings. We use our minds to judge by and do not hear what our feelings silently tell us. In developing our awareness of belonging to ourselves, we can awaken again the childhood sense of belonging to all of life and nature and the human family.

Body awareness can lead to larger, planetary awareness. Experiencing our sensual and emotional power enables us to respond with real compassion and caring to the sensate world around us, and to the feelings of others, without fear or reserve. Learning once more to unite body and mind, to trust ourselves to feel, and to "open up" to reality, can restore the confidence, and the ability to act and respond, that come from being truly in touch with ourselves.

"Members of a culture which is still totally contained in wilderness...have something which distinguishes them most strikingly from most people on this planet. It is a primal fact of existence, a dominant feeling, that no matter where they are known... they belong. In this world of ours we have lost this feeling of belonging."
Laurens van der Post

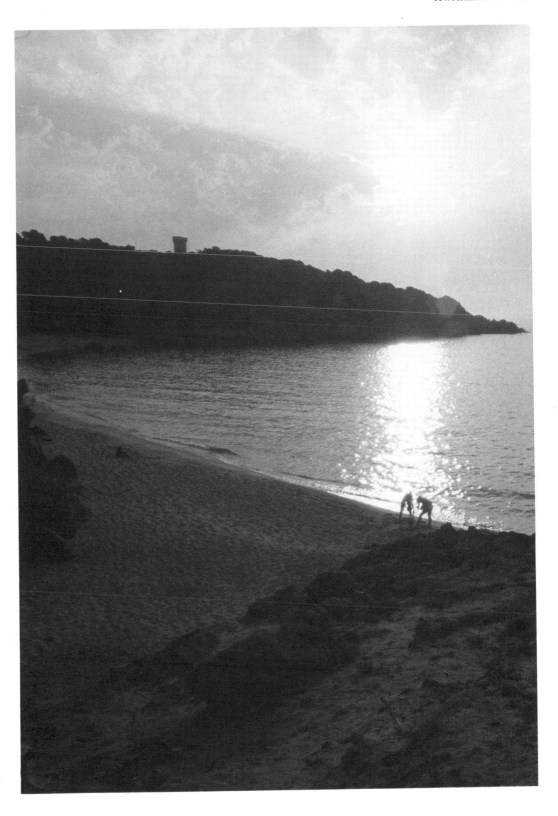

Appendix of bodymind therapies

As well as the techniques featured in this book, there are a number of other bodymind disciplines you might like to explore, that can enhance your vitality and self-awareness. Some of the most common disciplines are described below; others include techniques used mainly in group therapy, such as Gestalt and psychodrama, and body therapies, such as Rolfing. You can also extend the principles of body awareness outlined in this book to other forms of exercise and sport, provided you approach them with the right attitude, avoiding competitiveness and self-criticism, and keeping your attention on the sensations in your body.

Alexander technique

The Alexander technique is a way of relearning the skill we all had as young children: maintaining balance and poise with minimal tension. We "unlearn" our natural state when we react to stress by stiffening our necks or hunching our shoulders. By making unnecessary efforts to do even the simplest things, we drain our energy and often feel ill or beset with back pain. To counteract these tendencies, F. Matthias Alexander (1869-1955) developed a way of teaching conscious awareness of movement and posture. In a series of one-to-one sessions, the Alexander teacher observes you lying down, standing, sitting, and walking. As you move or pose, the teacher gently manipulates the muscles engaged, while giving you the appropriate directive (e.g. "neck free, head forward and out"). In allowing yourself to go with the new instruction, you also learn to "inhibit" your impulse to move in the old, distorted way. You will feel the point of perfect balance as a great lightness, and find that your movements flow easily into each other. By mentally directing your body to reach this point in all your everyday activities, you can gradually reclaim energies lost through tension and begin to really live in your body.

Biodynamic psychology

Biodynamic psychology is a holistic therapy, developed by Gerda Boyesen, which helps body and mind together to generate a healing process. Boyesen saw the libido or life force as the link between mind and body. She found that when the normally free-flowing libido is blocked by trauma, fluid builds up in our tissues, and emotions are stalled in our psyches, creating depression and anxiety. Boyesen also found that the intestines actually digest the stress from this pressure, and that a special form of massage can activate them and release the tension. In this technique, known as "psychoperistaltic massage", the therapist listens to your intestinal rumblings through a stethoscope as he or she massages different parts of your body. The release of the fluid – and the tension – can be heard in loud, distinct reports from the gut. By moving his or her hands just over your body, the therapist can harmonize the libido. In time this release allows you to integrate the repressed parts of yourself and begin to experience pleasure more fully.

Reichian bodywork

A one-time member of Freud's inner circle, Wilhelm Reich (1897-1958), broke away from the verbal approach of psychoanalysis to develop methods of liberating inhibitions by working with the body. He believed that we build up a rigid body "armour" of posture and facial expression by repressing our emotions and "forbidden" impulses. We can only be fully alive and emotionally healthy, he maintained, when we are able to free our life energy, or "orgone", and release it in emotional expression and through the orgastic reflex. In a typical session, you lie down and begin by breathing deeply. As you bring more energy into your body you will find you need to discharge it – usually as an outpouring of emotions. But often, your tensed muscles will dam this flow. The therapist will then carefully massage your muscles to help the release process.

Chi Kung

Chi Kung is a traditional Chinese healing system rooted in Taoism which, through breathing techniques, postures, movement, and meditation helps the student to harness *chi*, the life force around which Aikido and T'ai chi also centre. Its practice teaches you to balance *yin* and *yang*, the passive and active forces, so that *chi* flows freely, bringing you into harmony with yourself and the world. In Chi Kung you learn to follow four basic principles: relaxation, tranquillity, awareness, and motion. By first centering your awareness on the source of *chi*, below the navel, you learn to lower your rate of breathing, which increases lung capacity and clears the body of toxins. Gradually you begin to co-ordinate this new way of breathing with the Chi Kung postures and movement sequences. With dedicated application, you can achieve a state of freely flowing energy, expressed as a tranquil alertness, physical suppleness, and poise.

Dance

Dance is total, organic involvement; in freed movement we can get to know our bodies, express our inner selves and rediscover our sense of creativity. Early pioneers like Rudolph Laban and Margaret Morris recognized and promoted dance as a therapeutic activity for the ordinary person, sparking off a current of ideas that led to fresh ways of interpreting dance. Alain and Françoise Chantraine developed one such method, with the aim of "movement and dance as aids to the person". Their grounding in music, dance, art, psychology, and physiology led them to the belief that dance is life in concentrated form and that, as with all aspects of life, dance is most self-expressive when body, mind, and spirit are unified. In the classes, working at your own pace in a non-competitive atmosphere, you learn to relax and recharge and to replace self-criticism and tension with a new joy in movement.

Feldenkrais method

Designed by Dr. Moshe Feldenkrais, this method is a body-centered learning process in which both specific movement sequences and verbal guidance play a part. Aimed at correcting bad habits of body use and retraining the body into free and easy movement patterns, it combines a detailed scientific basis with a sense of gentle playfulness and curiosity. The method is taught in two formats: Awareness Through Movement (group classes) and Functional Integration (individual lessons). In a typical group session, the teacher guides you verbally through a variety of movements. Imaginative exercises, such as mentally scanning your body sensations, help in breaking up tensions. Functional Integration, which is best suited for those with special needs, incorporates light manipulation with these techniques. Both formats promote structural balance, easier breathing, and a sense of emotional well-being.

Meditation

Meditation is a method of training your awareness. By learning to reduce your mental chatter, you begin to reduce mental and physical tension and open your mind to calm and insight. To begin meditating effectively, you need to find a quiet room and set aside any expectations of what the meditation will bring you. There are many forms of meditation, both seated and active, spiritual and secular, but no particular belief is necessary for it to be effective. Methods of stilling the mind vary – among the most common are silently repeating a mantra, concentrating on a candle or other object, or focusing attention on your breathing.

Yoga

Yoga is the oldest system of mental, physical, and spiritual development in the world. Through its practice the individual self is allied with the absolute, or pure consciousness. Hatha Yoga, the one most commonly found in the West, is a complete mind-body science; it teaches mental discipline and concentration through which you can connect your body with conscious spirit. Breathing exercises (*pranayama*) and postures (*asanas*) are equally important parts of this process. In a typical yoga session, you practise *pranayama* before the *asanas* to purify your system, activate the flow of life energy (*prana*), and still the mind. You may also begin by adopting the Corpse pose, in which you lie on the floor and consciously relax each part of your body in turn. Your own needs and level of experience determine the *asanas* practised. Normally you practise a series of *asanas* in a session, each one counterbalancing the one before, so that the body is stretched equally in all directions. *Asanas* are performed slowly and with concentration and the positions are maintained for as long as possible.

Recommended Reading

Alexander, Gerda, *Eutony*, Felix Morrow, 1985
Barbach, Lonnie, *For Each Other*, Corgi, 1982
Brooks, Charles V. W., *Sensory Awareness*, Ross-Erikson, 1974
Csaky, Mick ed., *How does it feel?* Thames and Hudson, 1979
Dychtwald, Ken, *Body-Mind*, Jove Books, 1977
Ernst, Sheila and Goodison, Lucy, *In Our Own Hands*, The Women's Press, 1981
Huang, Al Chung-liang, *Embrace Tiger, Return to Mountain*, Real People Press, 1973
Johnson, Don, *Body*, Beacon Press, 1983
Keane, Betty Winkler, *Sensing*, Harper & Row, 1979
Kirsta, Alix, *The Book of Stress Survival*, Allen & Unwin, 1986, U.K., and Simon & Schuster, 1986, U.S.A.
Kripalu Center for Holistic Health, *The Self-Health Guide*, Kripalu Publications, 1980
Kurtz, Ron and Prestera, Hector M.D., *The Body Reveals*, Harper & Row, 1976
Lidell, Lucy, *The Book of Massage*, Ebury Press, 1984, U.K., and Simon & Schuster, 1984, U.S.A.
Lowen, Alexander M.D. and Lowen, Leslie, *The Way to Vibrant Health*, Harper Colophon, 1977
Lowen, Alexander M.D., *Bioenergetics*, Penguin, 1975
Macy, Joanna, *Personal Power in the Nuclear Age*, New Society Publishers, Philadelphia, 1973
Man-ch'ing, Cheng and Smith, Robert W., *T'ai chi*, Charles E. Tuttle, 1967
Man-ch'ing, Cheng, *T'ai chi Ch'uan*, North Atlantic Books, 1981
Montagu, Ashley, *Touching*, Harper Colophon, 1971
Rohé, Fred, *The Zen of Running*, Random House, 1974
Rosenberg, Jack Lee, *Total Orgasm*, Wildwood House, 1974
Rush, Anne Kent, *Getting Clear*, Wildwood House, 1974
Saito, Morihiro, *Aikido – its heart and appearance*, Minato research and publishing, 1975
Sivananda Yoga Centre, *The Book of Yoga* (with Lucy Lidell), Ebury Press, 1983, U.K., and *Sivananda Companion to Yoga*, Simon & Schuster, 1983, U.S.A.
Stanway, Andrew M.B., M.R.C.P., *The Natural Family Doctor*, Century Hutchinson, 1987, U.K., and Simon & Schuster, 1987, U.S.A.
Tulku, Tarthang, *Kum Nye Relaxation, parts 1 and 2*, Dharma Publishing, 1978
Ueshiba, Kisshomaru, *The Spirit of Aikido*, Kodansha International, 1984
Von Durckheim, Karlfried Graf, *Hara, The Vital Centre of Man*, Unwin Paperbacks, 1977

Useful Addresses

Body-centered psychotherapy, biodynamic massage, bioenergetics:
Chiron Centre
26 Eaton Rise
Ealing
London W5 2ER

Massage, healing, and psychotherapy:
Sara Thomas
15a Bridge Avenue
London W6

Psychotherapy, co-counselling:
Denis Postle
68a Church Road
Richmond
Surrey

Psychotherapy, sexuality counselling, and bodywork:
Spectrum
55 Dartmouth Park Road
London NW5 1SL

African dance:
Africa Centre
38 King Street
London WC2

Adzidzo African Dance Company
Duncombe Road
London N19

Eutony:
International association for Gerda Alexander eutony (AIEGA)
69 Rue du Rhône
CH-1207 Geneva

U.K.: Thérèse Melville-Van Cauwenberghe
68 Huntingdon Street
London N1

U.S.: Joyce Riveros
1633 Julian Drive
El Cerrito
CA 94530

Kum Nye, Chi Kung:
Franklin Sills
"Hopbines"
Eastington Cross
Lapford
Crediton
Devon EX17 6NE

Kum Nye:
U.S.: Nyingma Institute
1815 Highland Place
Berkeley
California
CA 94709

Aikido:
The London Aikido Club
4 Bath Street
London EC1

Yoga
Sivananda Yoga Vedanta Centre
50 Chepstow Villas
London W11

Index

Author's Acknowledgements

Many people helped to create this book. First of all, I would like to thank the contributors for enriching the project with their specialist knowledge: Frankie Armstrong, Thérèse Van Cauwenberghe, Barbara Karban, Peggy Harper, Denise Holmes, Denis Postle, Darien Pritchard, Franklin Sills, Sara Thomas, and Janaki Vincent. Several friends contributed much-appreciated advice on particular sections of the book: Jochen Lude on Breathing and Grounding; Janaki Vincent on Grounding; Anna Ickowitz on Rediscovering the Body; and Achim Korte on the Appendix. Special thanks also to: Barbara Karban for her beautiful watercolours; Pauline Hazelwood for her sensitive drawings; and Fausto Dorelli for his expressive photography; to Joss Pearson for her penetrating comments on the text; Susan Walby for so skilfully handling the book's production; Barbara Kiser for her work on the Appendix; and editor Susan McKeever and designer Peggy Sadler, a terrific team, for their patience, sensitivity, and understanding.

Many thanks also to: the Sivananda Yoga Centre for their generosity; Clive Lindley-Jones, Dr. A. R. Hibberd, and Jill Greeves for their support; Janet Wilkes for her kindness; Bernd Eiden, Hetty Einzig, and Thomas Dafferne for their advice; and Bob Moore, Hilmar Schönauer, and Andrew Watson, who inspired me to start my own personal quest. My deepest thanks are due to: my mother, Nancy Lidell, for her unfailing support; to Elaine Heller and Jane Downer, for their friendship, healing, and encouragement; and to Sara Thomas, whose collaboration and support throughout this project have been invaluable.

Gaia would like to extend thanks to the following:

Bolaji Adeola, Oriel and Paul Allsop, Simon Arnold, Barry Atkinson, Rod Birtles, Sue Brown, Imogen Bright, Michael Burman, Dijon Calew, Fausto Dorelli, Claire Duffett, Martha Fausset, Fred and Kathy Gill, Lesley Gilbert, Duncan Glass, David Hamilton, Pauline Hazelwood, Emer Heavey, Denise Holmes, Louise Jones, Barbara Karban, Barbara Kiser, Anna Kruger, Krishnabai, Venice Manley, all at Marlin Graphics, Chris McCorkindale, Ross McKelvie of Alfa Electronics, Erik Ness, Dave Nicholl, Melanie Nieuwenhuys, Nyingma Institute, On Yer Bike, Ruth O'Dowd, Lucy Oliver, Mary Perry, Kate Poole, Liz Renno, Sue Rose, Graeme Shawe, Franklin Sills, Sara Thomas, Arnold Udoka, Philippa Vine, Susan Walby, Peter Warren, Phil Wilkinson.

Photographic credits

All photographs in this book were taken by Fausto Dorelli, with the following exceptions:
p. 19 Ardea, London
pp. 21, 23, 25 Sally and Richard Greenhill
p. 27 Aspect Picture Library

Typesetting

Filmset in Sabon by Marlin Graphics Ltd., Orpington, Kent.

Colour reproduction

F.E. Burman Ltd., London